THE VIRTUOUS TART

RECIPES FREE FROM WHEAT,

DAIRY AND CANE SUGAR

RECIPES FREE FROM WHEAT, DAIRY AND CANE SUGAR

SUSAN JANE WHITE

GILL & MACMILLAN

GILL & MACMILLAN
Hume Avenue
Park West
Dublin 12
www.gillmacmillanbooks.ie

© Susan Jane White 2015

978 07171 6849 1

Designed by www.grahamthew.com

Photography © Joanne Murphy

Styled by Orla Neligan of Cornershop Productions: www.cornershopproductions.com

Assisted by Susie Coakley and Ross Murphy Cooke

Food prepared by Susan Jane White

Edited by Kristin Jensen

Indexed by Adam Pozner

Printed by L.E.G.O SpA

PROPS

Avoca: HQ Kilmacanogue, Bray, Co. Wicklow. T: (01) 2746939; E: info@avoca.ie;
W: www.avoca.ie

Meadows & Byrne: Dublin, Cork, Galway, Clare, Tipperary. T: (01) 2804554/
(021) 4344100; E: info@meadowsandbyrne.ie; W: www.meadowsandbyrne.com

Marks & Spencer: Unit 1-28, Dundrum Town Centre, Dublin 16. T: (01) 2991300;
W: www.marksandspencer.ie

Article Dublin: Powerscourt Townhouse, South William Street, Dublin 2.
T: (01) 6799268; E: items@articledublin.com; W: www.articledublin.com

Considered by Helen James, Dunnes Stores: 46-50 South Great Georges Street, Dublin
2. T: 1890 253185;
W: www.dunnesstores.com

Harold's Bazaar: 208 Harold's Cross Road, Dublin 6W. T: 087 7228789

Historic Interiors: Oberstown, Lusk, Co. Dublin. T: (01) 8437174;
E: killian@historicinteriors.net

TK Maxx: The Park, Carrickmines, Dublin 18. T: (01) 2074798; W: www.tkmaxx.ie

A.Rubanesque: T: (01) 6729243; E: ribbons@arubanesque.ie; W: arubanesque.ie

Tiger Stores: T: (01) 598 8800; W: tiger-stores.ie

The Patio Centre: The Hill Centre, Johnstown Road, Glenageary, Cabinteely,
Dublin 18. T: (01) 2350714; W: www.thepatiocentre.com

Industry Design: 41 A/B Drury Street, Dublin 2. T: (01) 6139111;
W: www.industrydesign.ie

This book is typeset in 9 on 11 point Botanika Mono Lite.

The paper used in this book comes from the wood pulp of managed forests. For every
tree felled, at least one tree is planted, thereby renewing natural resources.

A CIP catalogue record for this book is available from the British Library.

54321

ACKNOWLEDGEMENTS

THANK YOU

To my readers, without whom none of these crazy assed recipes could transpire. A heartfelt body slam.

To my sparkling team at Gill & Macmillan – Nicki Howard, Teresa Daly, Kristin Jensen, Catherine Gough and Paul Neilan. I do hope your adrenal glands are still on speaking terms with you. Your dedication is gobsmacking. A sincere thank you and *grá mór*.

To Brendan O'Connor and Mary O'Sullivan in the *Sunday Independent* for taking a chance on me all those years ago. By golly I'm grateful.

To my frontier of inspiration, Jamie Oliver, and his scorching team at Fresh One Productions. Especially you, JA.

To the Snazz Meister, Graham Thew, whose brilliance is peerless.

To photographer Jo Murphy and stylist Orla Neligan, two fireflies behind the lens. To megassistants Susie and Ross, for their tireless enthusiasm and blessed Marigolds.

To dearest Saskia Vermeulen, it's a privilege to work with such talent and tenacity.

Rascals one and two: your courage to sample everything Mummy makes is, well, alarming. You rock.

To my mother Olive, an excellent role model who only ever sees the positive things in life. Like turning burnt cake into exotic granola. And making my lips a feature to distract from my flat chest.

A final and thunderous thanks goes to my fearless (self-appointed) editor-in-chief, TW. You drive me bonkers. (In a good way.)

CONTENTS
+++++++

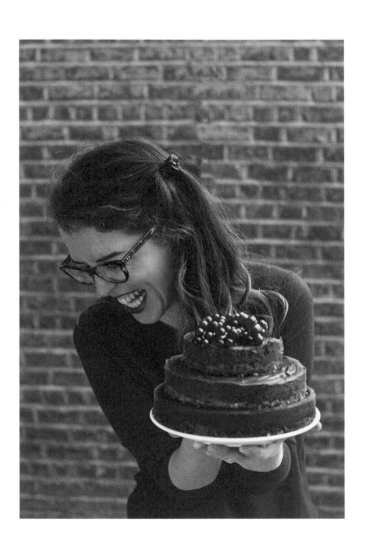

INTRO-
DUCTION

'A man who gives little time to health
will one day give much time to illness.'

WHAT'S IT ALL ABOUT?

Healthy food is all very well and good, but it's got to taste great, right? Damn right! I love cooking for flavour, but cooking for the good of my body makes me giddy. **It's like dating a terribly tasty hunk, then finding out he's rich too**.

Health and flavour are my thing, a potent duo. This way of cooking stokes the imagination. Gives wings to your spice rack. Thrills the body. And places vitality at the centre of your table.

Imagine a nutritional slam-dunk while snacking on a slice of tiffin. Picture your taste buds raving to the tune of BBQ veg crisps or your toes break dancing with every crunch and snap of a teff cookie. Wholesome food need never tax your taste buds.

Food is information. Every bite we eat contains software that tells our genes how to express themselves. Food literally has the ability to turn our 'good' genes on and our 'bad' genes off. By nourishing your body with the right nutrients, your body will nourish you. **It makes a lot of sense to count nutrients, not calories**. If calorie-controlled diets worked, we'd all be thin (and achingly dull).

So what counts as nourishing? Raw, unprocessed food like whole fruit, quirky beans, fresh vegetables, groovy grains such as buckwheat and quinoa, and weird-sounding flours milled from chickpeas and rye. Fat is your friend: chia, olive, flaxseed, almonds, avocados, oily fish and coconut. These choices will service your body like a first-rate Formula 1 pit stop, and you'll have the winning body to prove it. Whether it's in the boardroom, college library or on the track, we want to perform, right? Let's not sabotage our own fuel supply.

Yet that's exactly what I did 10 years ago. I thought I was too busy to cook and cycled past my local grocer, cackling at the queues. **Turns out smarter people make time to cook. Smarter people pay the grocer, not the doctor**. Smarter people embrace cooking as an adventure, a love affair. Smarter people prioritise their health over their wristwatch. The irony was rather spectacular.

It wasn't wheat, sugar or dairy that triggered my portfolio of health disorders. It was the industrial amount of it I was consuming and the dodgy expiry dates that accompanied my preferred junk foods. I thought healthy food was for the elderly or infirm. I convinced myself that pepperoni was a

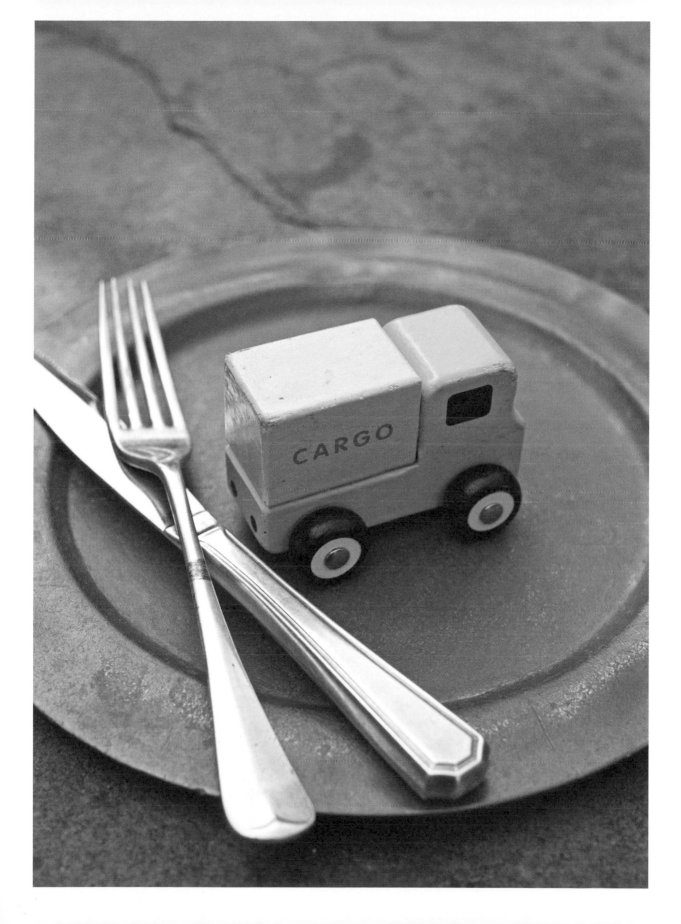

vegetable. I counted coffee as one of my five a day (coffee beans are from a plant, right?) and horsed into breakfast cereals with a misguided sense of passion normally only seen in Silvio Berlusconi.

Eventually my body said no. Enough. First up was chronic stomach upsets that felt, and sounded, like a civil war was erupting inside my colon. Then exhaustion, with no energy to think straight, to make judicious decisions, to summon patience when required. Then insomnia set in and symptoms rocketed as I dragged my body around campus thinking it was quite acceptable to feel ill and confused in my twenties. My peers weren't the epitome of health either, but it was difficult to tell hangovers apart from deeper health issues. One thing was clear, though: we were digging our way to the grave with our teeth.

The amount of white flour, white sugar and dairy we eat is borderline pathological. Cereal and milk for breakfast, sandwiches for lunch, scones, cake, toast, biccies, pasta - the same old circus day in, day out. Sound familiar? My body begged for a break. Maybe yours is screaming for one too.

I'm not against wheat, sugar and dairy. They're all delightfully alluring. But my energy levels are a whole lot better when I cut back on their mindless consumption. When I open up my food choices to all the other exhilarating ingredients around me, suddenly I find that eating less wheat, less sugar and less dairy isn't restrictive at all. In fact, it's the exact opposite. My choices become liberated and I discover loads of fabulous stuff I didn't even know existed.

We are excluding so many outrageously tasty foods when we're stuck in the dairy-wheat-sugar love triangle. Are you a fan of crisps? Wait until you try them made from Jerusalem artichokes! You think I'm joking? Just turn to page 129. Fudge brownies? They're way better made with sticky dates and walnuts. Love pasta and couscous? Not when you discover at least a dozen tastier choices in the Asian supermarket, ranging from black sticky rice to mung bean noodles.

Figure out what makes your body feel good. Pizza, ice cream and soda can be like a two-faced friend who's kind to your face, then stabs you in the back. So thrill the bejaysus out of your taste buds. Spicy black bean chilli? Raw chocolate torte? Maple and sesame halva? Now you're listening. That was your body talking. Work with your appetite instead of fearing it. You already know what your body needs.

WHY SUGAR FREE?

I used to carry Kit Kats like cigarettes. An expert sugar junkie.

Not anymore. I've cut out nasty refined sugar and ditched sodas. This simple change has transformed my energy levels and even my dress size. And guess what? It's far from restrictive, which was my first assumption when I embarked on this crazy-assed plan. It's the exact opposite.

Suddenly I found loads of different ingredients within my orbit that not only tasted better, but treated my body better too. Discoveries included chestnut flour, Medjool dates, coconut sugar and naturally sweet spices like cinnamon and liquorice. These flavours helped nurse my sweet tooth while recalibrating my taste buds.

It's science, innit? My taste buds have been reprogrammed. Yours will be too. Along with this reprogramming comes a profound sense of respect for my body and how it works. That's because every bite I took affected my mood, my skin and my energy, either positively or negatively.

I'm not controlled by the sugar highs anymore. I have escaped their poxy shackles. Ever known what it's like to be in the nucleus of a comet? This might be your year.

So how can you **service your cravings and lessen the damage**? Look at Mother Nature's stash of nectar (turn the page). All contain valuable trace minerals and vitamins as well as offering that sensual sweet hit - Ray LaMontagne on the lips.

If your diet obliges you to stay off sugar, this means quarantining all forms of sugar, good *and* bad, from your diet, including maple syrup, honey and even dried fruit. My cookbook only evicts nasty white sugar from your kitchen. **I can't accuse any sugar of being nutritious, but what follows is my list of healthier choices** when it comes to tickling a sweet tonsil. Glycemic loads, per serving, are scribbled to the side for diabetics to note. As with all sugars, you can pack on the pounds if you're using them with glorious abandon. Think of these as sweet treats. If sugar, even natural ones, becomes a staple in your kitchen, you'll have the waistline to prove it!

Candida diets require the elimination of *all* sugars, including natural, unprocessed sugars like fresh fruit. Small amounts of stevia and xylitol are permissible, but it's always a good idea to find a specialist to embark on this candida pilgrimage with you. You'll slowly be able to reintroduce natural sugars to your diet, mindfully, just like I did.

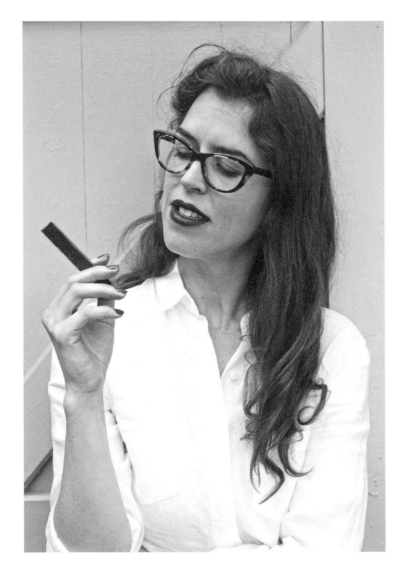

*'I used to carry Kit Kats like cigarettes.
An expert sugar junkie.'*

AGAVE (LOW GL) --

Agave syrup doesn't excite me, but it's still there on my shelf.

So what's the deal with this fructose syrup? Fructose is a naturally occurring sugar found in fruit and some veg, but in small concentrations. It's also delivered alongside the other minerals and fibre contained within that piece of fruit. When fructose is artificially concentrated, like when agave is manufactured, and in isolation from other nutrients, our body treats it quite differently. Glucose is metabolised by every cell in the body, says endocrinologist Dr Robert Lustig. Fructose, however, can only be metabolised by the liver. Too much fructose in a concentrated, isolated form has been shown to burden the liver.

Much of the research on high fructose corn syrup (HFCS) exposes its adverse health effects, especially in the form of liquids. Drinks and confectionary sweetened with HFCS shoot excessive amounts of concentrated fructose to the liver, the outcome of which is more than alarming. For more on this, I recommend reading authors Dr Robert Lustig, Michael Moss and Marion Nestle.

I think agave can be useful in small quantities for diabetics as an occasional treat. Diabetics have it tough. Honey, maple syrup, dried fruit, date syrup - all are delisted for the diabetic. The alternative for diabetics is xylitol (not a fan), stevia (never liked it) or artificial sweeteners (no chance). In this light, agave has a functional and positive use in the kitchen as long as you don't stick a straw in the bottle and neck the lot.

BARLEY MALT SYRUP (LOW-MEDIUM GL) ---------------------------

This licky-sticky yummy stuff is responsible for the taste of Maltesers, barbeque sauce, bagels and beer. What's not to love? Barley malt syrup has great attitude in the kitchen. It's half as sweet as honey but twice as thick, so don't substitute it one for one in recipes. This might explain why so few celebrity chefs use it. One diva in the kitchen is already too much.

Production of barley malt syrup is peculiar. This rich caramel is made by soaking and germinating barley to activate important enzymes - a process often referred to as malting. The sprouted grain is then dried before it's cooked slowly at a low temperature. I imagine the smell is delightfully inebriating. The resulting ambrosial liquid is strained of any impurities and sent to stores in glass jars.

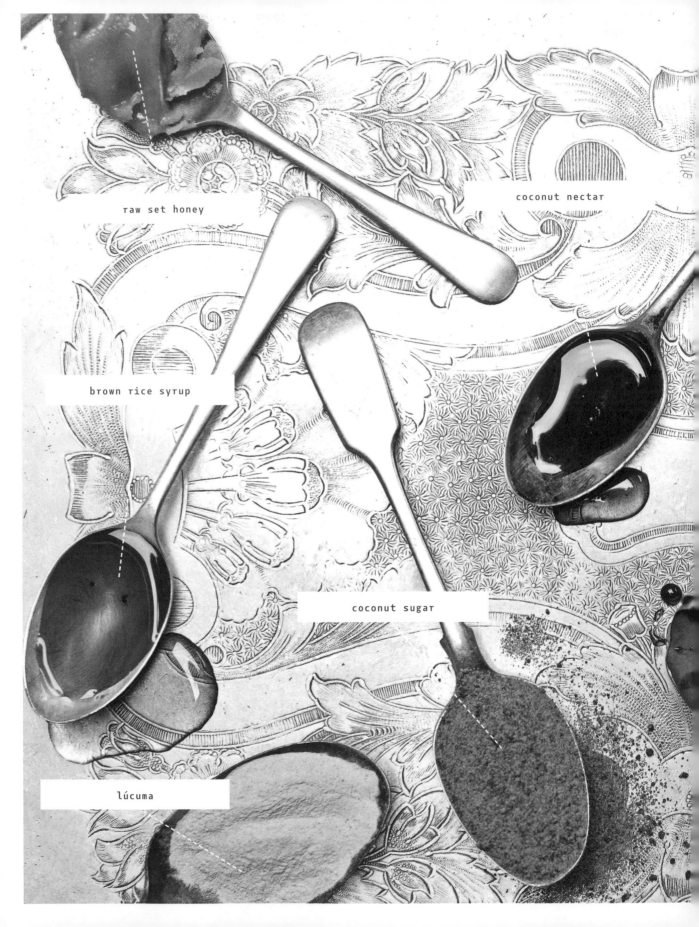

raw set honey

coconut nectar

brown rice syrup

coconut sugar

lúcuma

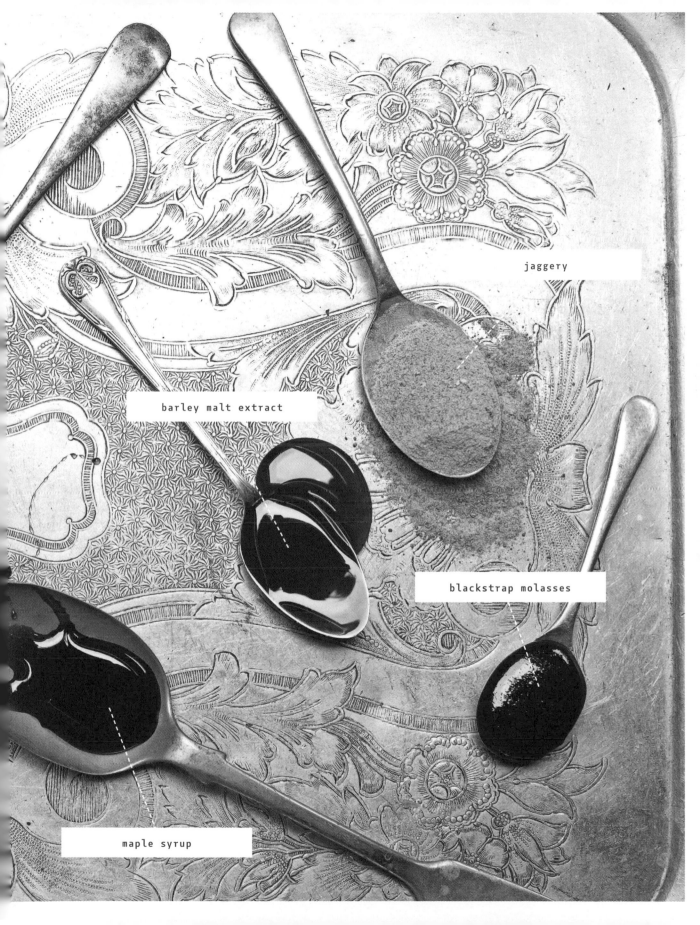

BLACKSTRAP MOLASSES (MEDIUM GL) ----------------------------

Molasses is that earthy sweetness found partying in gingerbread and baked beans. This incredulously sticky syrup is closer to tar than sugar cane. At less than 1 cent per gram, it's a fairly sweet deal too.

Black molasses is the syrup that's left over from the process of turning sugar cane into table sugar. The plant's nutrients are concentrated in its juice, then boiled and boiled into a fudgy molasses. Unlike table sugar, artificial sweeteners or fructose syrups, blackstrap molasses is humming with a variety of minerals that help promote good health. But don't squeal yet - it's not the new coconut nectar. Black molasses is only a fraction as sweet as regular sugar, imparts a mineral flavour that can be an acquired taste and can frequently misbehave in dishes. More often than not, it's just misunderstood. Once you get to know it better, you'll find its inadequacies charming and much easier to work with.

For a sugar, blackstrap molasses is a surprisingly good source of iron (useful for vegetarians or incorrigibly moody teens). Without sufficient iron, our bodies struggle to make haemoglobin. This is the stuff that helps transport oxygen around our system. No oxygen, no mojo. Sound familiar, ladies? That's because iron deficiency is more common in women than in men. One tablespoon of blackstrap molasses also shoots us with 15% of our recommended calcium intake, making jam warble with envy. Breathless yet?

BROWN RICE SYRUP (LOW-MEDIUM GL) ----------------------------

Apparently brown rice syrup is soaked in symbolism. It stands for more than just a sweetener. Ever heard of Russell Brand? Joaquin Phoenix? Jared Leto? All are indecently hunky-looking vegans who prefer brown rice syrup to honey. Brown rice syrup says, 'I am kind. I am sweet. I am savvy.' So I signed up.

Despite brown rice syrup being a fairly processed product, it has low levels of glucose (about 5%) and high levels of the more complex carbohydrate maltose (around 55%). This gives it an attractive glycemic load that drip-feeds your body's battery. Table sugar has a high glycemic load, giving you explosive bursts of energy but leaving you with a sugar hangover and often a greater deficit in energy than before the initial hit.

Brown rice syrup is made by fermenting the cooked grain with cultured enzymes to break down its carbohydrates. The liquid by-product is boiled to make sweet, sticky syrup. It can come in a variety of 'processed' gradients worthy of further sleuthing. Sticking to organic seems sensible given the volume of agrichemicals regularly used in rice production. For example, a few years back there was some alarm regarding arsenic levels in brown rice and apples from particular parts of the world. Keep those antennae finely tuned.

CINNAMON (LOW GL) ---

This warming spice is naturally very sweet and doesn't tax blood sugar levels. There is considerable hype about cinnamon's ability to control diabetes, but these are premature claims, I'm afraid. There is insubstantial evidence to date, or at least none significant enough to merit such accolades. But it tastes great in baked goods, hot chocolate and porridge, so go ahead and parachute it onto your goodies as a natural source of sweetness.

COCONUT BLOSSOM SYRUP (LOW GL) -----------------------------

See coconut sugar. The syrup is less heat treated than crystallised coconut sugar. The only brands I have found in the UK and Ireland are Biona and Coconut Secret (which does a splendiferous raw version). Let me know when more brands come on the market where you live - send me a tweet @SusanJaneHealth #extravirginkitchen.

COCONUT SUGAR (LOW GL) -------------------------------------

In 2014 I flicked coconut blossom sugar out of my cupboard, condemning it as another hysterical trend for the kale-gnawing postcodes of London. But somehow it slipped back under my radar and spectacularly high-jumped my cynicism. Now I like to look at my packet of coconut palm sugar and stroke it like an adorable little sea urchin.

Think granulated toffee. Crunchy caramel. Got it? Coconut nectar doesn't have that sickly sweet kick of regular sugar, which does frightening things to my heartbeat. Too good to be true?

Here's what happens in far-off places like Bali, king of the coconut community. Nectar from the coconut palm tree is collected by securing a vessel underneath the tree's flowers to collect its sticky sap. This liquid nectar is then roasted in big cauldrons to boil off the water content and turn it into a sweet, viscous syrup. To make a crystallised sugar, the syrup is boiled some more and left to cool before massaging and grinding it into granules. Many small boutique producers in Bali will sieve the sugar to create a fine, powdery coconut palm sugar for the Western market, but locals will use it in big clumsy clumps. Coconut nectar and coconut sugar are unlike any other sweeteners I have tasted: smooth like caramel, yet acidic and fruity. Lip-smackingly fabulous. The finished product is a whole sweetener, which means its nutrition is intact and hasn't been stripped away. Don't get me wrong – coconut sugar is still a sugar, like all these natural sweeteners, but it's a less evil variety. You'll find surprising amounts of iron and potassium in coconut sugar, which may help explain why athletes become curiously giddy at the mere mention of it. But this sweetener's USP is its low glycemic range. Coconut sugar won't spike your blood sugar levels and leave you with a crashing low that ultimately drives the vicious circle of craving more sugar and another high.

DATE SYRUP (MEDIUM-HIGH GL) -----------------------------------

These wondrous fruits frequently disrupt my sleep. When I know I have a bag of sticky Medjool dates downstairs, it's almost traumatic to keep my mind and mitts off them. Try eating one without levitating.

These delectable dried fruits contain modest amounts of alkalising minerals such as potassium, magnesium and calcium. Dates can be alchemised into a paste or syrup by boiling different varieties and reducing the liquid to a viscose treacle. Date syrup has a higher glycemic value than other sweeteners, making it desirable for gym bunnies. However, this also means that date syrup is off limits for diabetics, as it can fiddle with blood sugar levels. While dates aren't fattening, overindulging will force the body to store its excess sugars with your fat depot. So munch in moderation unless an afternoon with Rich Roll and Brendan Brazier is planned.

JAGGERY (MEDIUM GL) ---

Jaggery comes from 70-foot-high Palmyra palms. The nectar of the fruit is collected, gently heated and then dehydrated to become an irresistible powdery sweetener. White sugar is boring, predictable and bankrupt in comparison. Like an ex, you'll wonder what you ever saw in it.

This caramel-coloured dust imparts a rich flavour to baked goodies, similar to molasses. It has a desirable low-medium glycemic load and only tiny amounts of fructose (if this concerns you). Deep, dark, musky and sticky – all the virtues required of a naughty treat. But iron? And B vitamins? There's the thunderbolt.

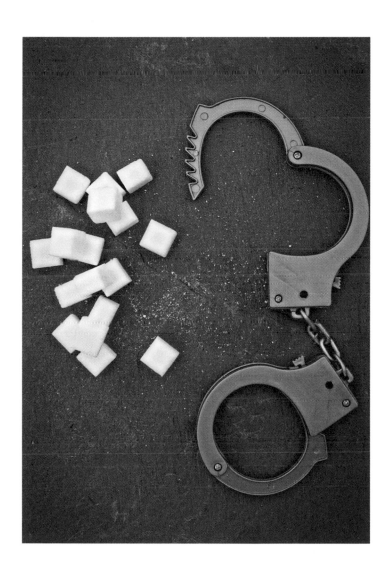

B vitamins help your battery, your body and your brain (and don't forget B for bad hangover). Stress robs your bank of B vitamins. If you run out of your B supply, your body will struggle to make stress-related hormones, nourish nerves or watch *House of Cards* without your adrenal glands combusting. Stress, then, creates a need for vitamins to be replaced. Often we reach for Marlboros and lattes, when all your body needs is a wholesome meal to get you cantering again.

It's probably better if you nosedive into a bowl of quinoa or run up some buckwheat pancakes for your hit of B vitamins, but during your hour of need, when faced with a packet of candy or the prospect of a hot Honut (page 146) or MILF Muffin (page 86) in less than 20 minutes, I'd like to think I helped you make the finer decision.

LIQUORICE (LOW GL) --

Like cinnamon, liquorice is another naturally sweet spice that can be used to serenade that sweet tooth. I put it in the Apple and Winter Squash Crumble on page 150 for Christmas.

LÚCUMA (LOW GL) --

You can find lúcuma in powdered form on the shelves of savvy grocers and health stores. A spoonful of this silky smooth Peruvian fruit is enough to incite poetry in AA Gill. Dried lúcuma is a scrumptious way of naturally sweetening dishes while providing niacin - aka vitamin B3 - to help the crusade against cholesterol and depression. Lúcuma's iron and beta-carotene content should also help stoke your immunity. A toughie to find in stores, order lúcuma powder online or through your local health food store. It's insanely expensive, so I use it as a flavour rather than a straight-up sweetener.

MAPLE SYRUP (MEDIUM GL) --

Maple syrup is a gloriously rich sweetener. The syrup hails from the concentrated sap of maple trees, which retains surprising amounts of iron and calcium. Grade B maple syrup is considered superior. Maple syrup is one of the few sweeteners (alongside date syrup) that leave an alkaline footprint. Other sugars can be highly acidic to the system, especially cane sugar. Acidity has been shown to leach calcium from bones, while alkaline diets enhance calcium absorption. This is useful information if you suffer from arthritic and osteo conditions. But if you can do the Macarena without wincing, you're probably okay. Make the switch and see how you feel.

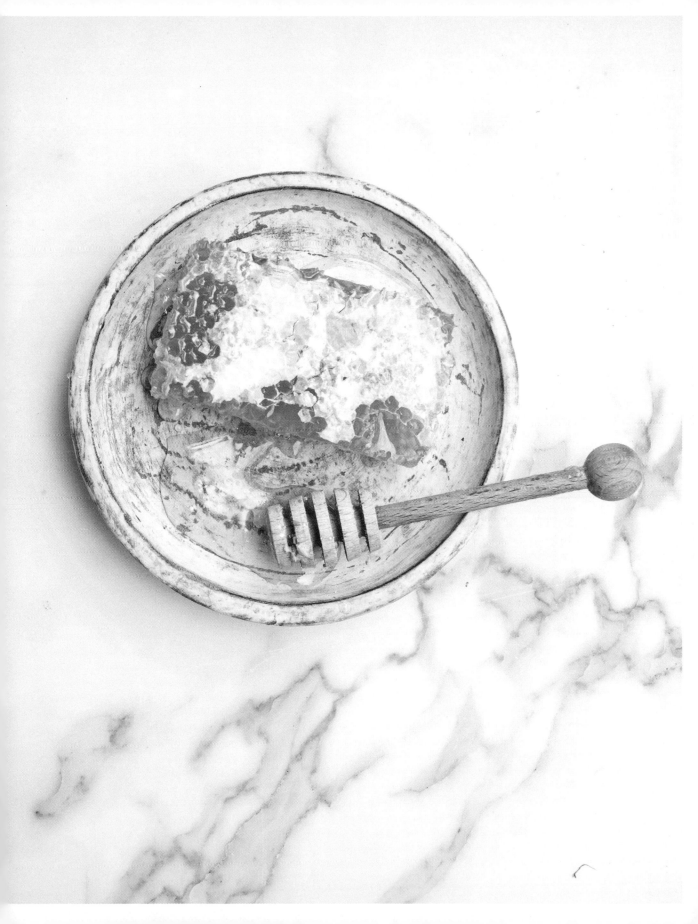

RAW HONEY (MEDIUM GL) --

Raw, local honey might sound a little bombastic, but I have a sense it's already in your cupboard. (Tara Hill honey from Wexford? Killarney Clover?) Local means you're high-fiving your town's economy as well as escaping industrial heat treatments that can diminish the honey's excitement. Just ask your regular health store to point out the local ones and taste the difference.

Hay fever veterans swear by it. Local honey contains manageable amounts of pollen from your postcode in it to prepare you for the sneezy season. There's immune-boosting propolis too and some serious antiviral, antifungal and antibacterial artillery.

How is it made? Female bees collect nectar from various plants, shrubs, trees and flowers, turning it into an alchemist's dream. Using special enzymes (that's diplomatic speak for frothy gob), the nectar turns into liquidy honey and is housed symmetrically in honeycomb. Then the bee dance begins (as illustrated in my toddler's Dr Seuss book). The female honeybees flap their wings with a fervour usually reserved for an underage Limerick rave. This dance helps to evaporate the water content from the nectar and turn it into the licky-sticky elixir as we know it.

'Honeycomb is altogether miraculous,' says Sarah Britton, founder of My New Roots. 'To behold its sheer geometrical perfection is like a religious experience, and to see evidence of the deep, clear intelligence that built such a structure is humbling.' Raw honey is very special – certainly one of life's greatest pleasures, along with itching, sneezing and submitting to chilli.

Commercial manuka honey can be subjected to intense heat treatment, making it somewhat controversial. Maddening, right? This honey hails from New Zealand's manuka foliage, which is thought to have particularly high antimicrobial properties. I find raw local honey more potent than most commercial brands of manuka. If you can get raw manuka, then lucky you! Applied topically, manuka honey has shown promising results in treating MRSA sores. It's worth remembering that you shouldn't cook with manuka honey either. This special type of honey prefers an empty belly for its health benefits to kick in.

STEVIA (ZERO GL) --

Stevia is so fashionable that MAC is naming a lipstick after it. (Okay, I made that up.)

Stevia can be purchased in liquid, crystallised, Erylite or powdered form. It's sweeter than white sugar, requires no insulin from your body to break it down and has no calories or nutrients. I'm not a fan, but I can understand why diabetics love it.

Interestingly, there is some controversy over stevia's ability to trick your mind into thinking you're eating sugar. Some health experts argue that this 'trick' is just as damaging to your blood sugar levels and your health, triggering hypoglycaemia in frequent users. But I don't imagine this would happen when kept to occasional treats, like the American Peanut Butter Cookies (page 137) or Limonade (page 78).

Stevia's peppermint chill gives a weird extraterrestrial vibe to baked goods. You'll love it or chuck it.

XYLITOL (VERY LOW GL) --
I prefer the term 'birch sugar' rather than xylitol, which sounds like a bunion buster. This relatively new sweetener is now available in health food stores and select pharmacies. I'm not convinced the processing is 'natural', but this hasn't stopped its roaring rise.

The sugar is mainly made by boiling birch sap until viscous and adding several curious chemicals to help the process. Judging by the brands available in our stores, my raised eyebrows note that some are industrially synthesised in labs using corn instead of birch, and details are shaky about their origin. Worthy of further sleuthing? Watch out for piracy too. New-fangled fads attract trouble like a pedigree Chihuahua in heat.

Children's confectionery brands are also turning towards xylitol. There is some noise about the reduction of bacterial growth in the mouth after the consumption of xylitol relative to cane sugar and dried fruit. The idea, then, is that xylitol may help reduce cavities - but so would reducing fizzy cola consumption or remembering to scrub your nashers more often. I'm keeping an open mind given its popularity among diabetics and health bloggers, but it ain't sharing a place with maple syrup in my kitchen.

Trouser trumpets (that's Latin for flatulence) and intestinal discomfort are an expected side effect for quantities that exceed the recommended daily intake. Many diabetics and weight watchers love xylitol, and sales figures show this. It's important to make up your own mind about it.

In theory, white sugar and xylitol can be interchanged without any mathematical gymnastics, which is good news for diabetics. In practice, it's a total queen. Xylitol can make a cake surprisingly crumbly, like the bottom of a box of Rice Krispies. If you fancy yourself a culinary MacGyver, you'll love the challenge of whipping it into submission. If not, I've alchemised a stonking good granola recipe on page 171 to get you started.

YACÓN SYRUP (LOW GL) ---------------------------------------

Known as the apple of the earth because of its inherent sweetness, this tuber vegetable makes wonderfully sticky syrup. Yacón nectar is definitely the nearest thing to golden syrup for health-conscious, smoothie-swilling folk.

Despite the unfortunate onomatopoeic ring to its name, yacón is in fact outlandishly tasty while magically low in calories and glycemic load. Hurrah! This is because of yacón's naturally high content of inulin, a complex sugar that breaks down very slowly in the body.

This food's trump card? Much of its inulin content will convert to fructooligosaccharides - that's doctor speak for prebiotics. Fructooligosaccharides make for happy bowels by feeding the good bacteria in our digestive tracts. Prebiotics are necessary for *probiotics* to multiply - in other words, better colon health.

Yacón is both pricey and tricky to source. See page 200 in the resources section for some leads.

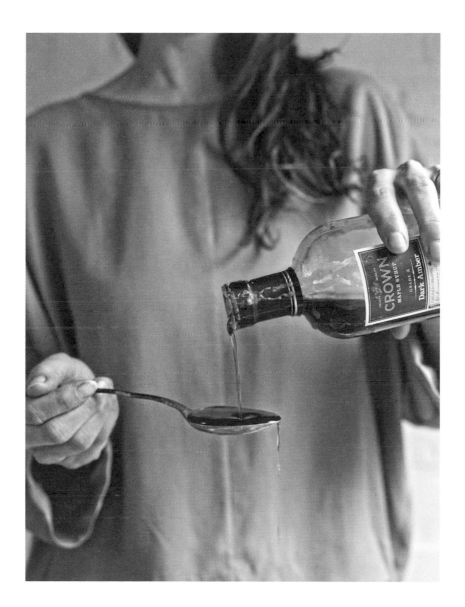

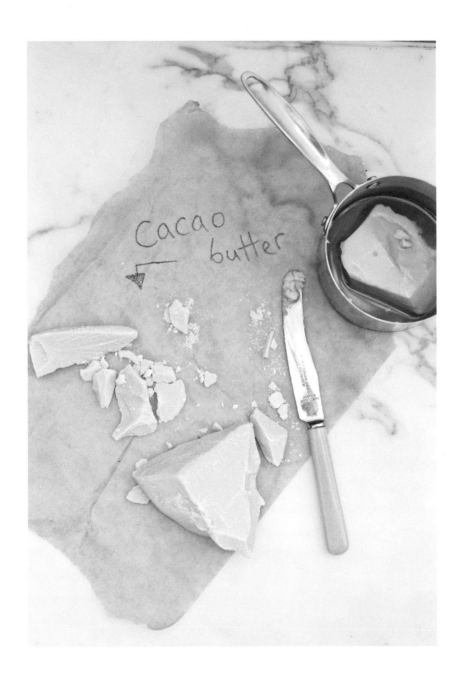

WHY DAIRY FREE?

What's this cowspiracy? Dairy - friend or foe? Both! My mate Oscar Wilde caught it best when he said 'everything in moderation, even moderation itself'. **There's nothing wrong with dairy. It's the sheer volume we consume that alarms me**.

The obsession with having dairy at every meal and its mindless consumption is causing problems in our diet. Too much of any type of food is bound to have negative consequences. Imagine if you ate turkey for breakfast, turkey slices as snacks, then turkey soup for lunch, followed by minced turkey for dinner and all washed down with turkey sambos. You'd think I was right-on bonkers. There's something pathologically queer about that diet, right? But that's what I was doing with dairy 10 years ago - I had milk and butter at every breakfast, yoghurt and smoothies as snacks, cheese sambos for lunch and creamy pasta for dinner. See? No wonder my body objected. We are suffering from a perverse form of dietary obsessive compulsory disorder to have dairy every day, and in some cases, several times a day. **Your body needs to samba to other nutrient-rich ingredients too**. The dairy industry and lazy dieticians will purport that dairy is an essential part of a balanced diet. But therein lies the problem! **Our diet is far from balanced**. Dairy has tipped the scales.

Let's be honest - the mindless consumption of wheat and sugar is facing the same problem. That's why I wrote this book. Let's get jiggy with some exciting new ingredients to hotwire our batteries and our bodies.

Other sources of calcium include tinned sardines and wild salmon (their bones are soft when canned and are wonderfully rich in calcium), soaked or sprouted almonds, hazelnuts, chia seeds, sesame and tahini, figs, chickpeas and hummus, barley grass powder, green leafy veg and sea veg. The proper absorption of calcium is a complicated biological process, one which modern science hasn't cracked. If we had nailed calcium's conundrum, why is our rate of osteoporosis so high? And our rate of hip fractures even higher than that of Japan's, where they don't even eat dairy?

Contrary to popular belief, a low intake of calcium isn't the primary cause of osteoporosis. The standard Western diet causes much of the consumed calcium to be lost in the urine, explains Dr Joel Fuhrman. 'Excess salt, caffeine, sugar, and animal products leach calcium out of bones and promote urinary calcium loss. The Nurses' Health Study followed 72,337 women for over 18 years and found that dairy intake did not reduce the risk of osteoporosis-related hip fractures.' It's not a simple matter, so don't be hoodwinked by those who tell you otherwise. It's worth doing your own research if this is an important area for you and your health. The Harvard School of Public Health is a good starting point.

I should point out that many other health advocates would outright reject dairy in the diet. **I'm not that extreme, but I'm happy to outline their reasons for doing so if it helps you understand the dairy-free movement.**

1. <u>Dairy contains a naturally occurring sugar called lactose</u>, which cannot be tolerated by those who do not make the special enzyme lactase to break it down in their body. For example, many Asians don't produce lactase. Science, innit?

2. Vegans reject dairy because it <u>exploits animals</u>. Grand so.

3. Some people <u>react to casein</u>, a protein found in milk. They will typically experience adverse effects when dairy is consumed and are likely to avoid milk in order to avoid the intestinal discomfort and drama. Nuff said.

4. <u>Goat's milk, while still 'dairy', is easier to digest</u>, especially for infants. This possibly gives cow's milk a bad rep by proxy.

5. The <u>use of antibiotics in dairy farming</u> is more than unattractive. Antibiotic residues are thought to transfer to the milk, and subsequently to the consumer. Massive industrial dairy farms, particularly in the US, treat the animals as horrific engines. Hygiene is dubious, which helps explain the extreme heat treatment to sterilise particles of infected puss found in some of the milk. This is what happens in massive dairy factories where cows are excessively milked and badly treated. These conditions are gruesome and unnatural. I'm confident that Irish milk escapes such barbaric treatment, but I promised to outline the main arguments in the dairy-free movement, so there you have it. Choose organic milk products from smaller dairy farms that take pride in the health of their herd, such as Ardmore, Glenilen and Glenisk. They need our support, so vote with your wallet.

6. The unnecessary <u>OD-ing on one food group</u> (see my introduction above).

7. Milk is, after all, <u>boob juice</u> from a stranger. Would you take your neighbour's breast milk? If not, ask yourself why a random bovine creature doesn't repel you. It's a good point, usually made by vegans. I'm not entirely put off dairy, but I find myself challenged by this particular sentiment. I'd rather have the taste of homemade almond milk any day, but I tremble at the thought of rejecting a cheese board at a fancy restaurant.

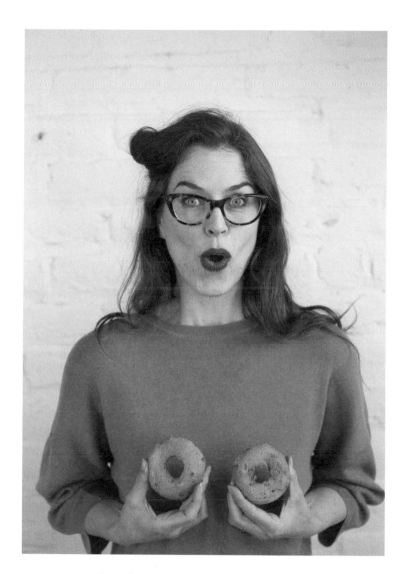

See Honuts recipe on p.146.

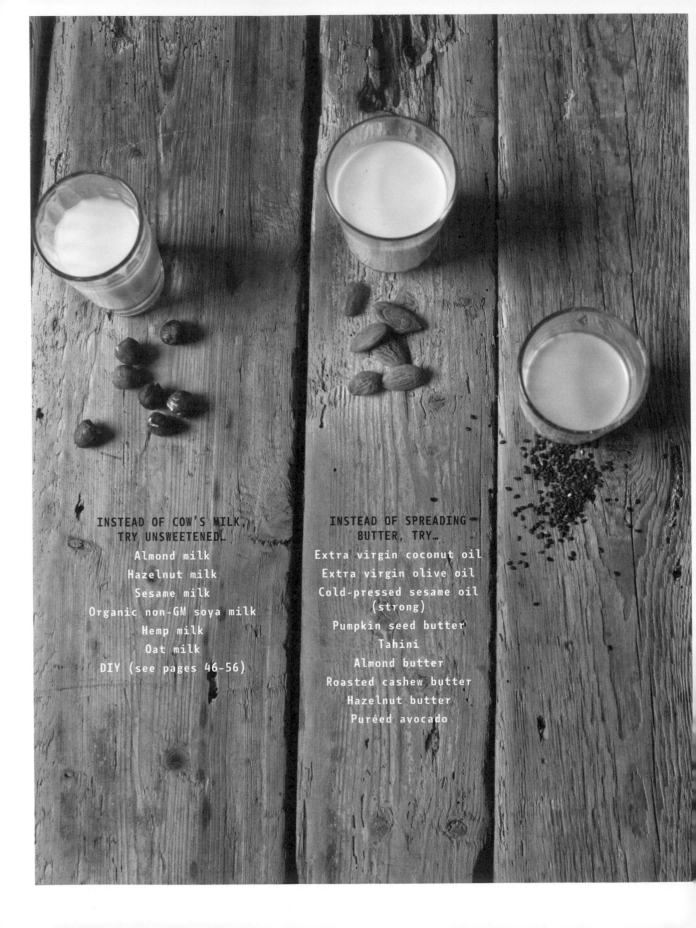

INSTEAD OF COW'S MILK,
TRY UNSWEETENED...

Almond milk

Hazelnut milk

Sesame milk

Organic non-GM soya milk

Hemp milk

Oat milk

DIY (see pages 46-56)

INSTEAD OF SPREADING
BUTTER, TRY...

Extra virgin coconut oil

Extra virgin olive oil

Cold-pressed sesame oil
(strong)

Pumpkin seed butter

Tahini

Almond butter

Roasted cashew butter

Hazelnut butter

Puréed avocado

THE BIG FAT CONTROVERSY ------------------------------------

Our relationship with fat is perverse. Some people are downright scared of it. I'm not one of them. Did you know that there are fats that heal and fats that harm?

Omega-3 fats are to hormones what Dolce is to Gabbana: intimately co-dependent. The endocrine system is like the call centre for hormones. It appears to rely heavily on the regular consumption of these essential fats from our diet. What happens when we don't get enough of these delicious fats in our diet? According to the scientific literature, our risk of presenting with mental health problems increases – depression, Alzheimer's, dementia, bipolar. Improved levels of omega-3 consumption can often form the basis of a recovery plan in many medical clinics. Omega-3s, particularly EPA and DHA, are by far the best researched and documented of the dietary fats. Diets rich in these fatty acids demonstrate some of the most wide-reaching health benefits, and they're not exclusive to brain development and Sudoku skills. They include improved heart health and immune function support, reduced risk of stroke and the ability to referee inflammation in the body better than any other fat.

The 'fat is evil' mantra is utterly bankrupt in the face of current nutritional science. Fat is not the enemy. If it was, then why are we getting fatter and fatter every year when the consumption of low-fat products has never been so popular?

It's what we do with fat that matters.

Nasty hydrogenating techniques plague our supermarket shelves, and consequently our waistlines and liver. These techniques lead to a gross degradation of the original fat, giving birth to what we now refer to as trans fats.

Food manufacturers love trans fats for their shelf life and low cost. Of course they do! But our arteries and livers clearly don't. You'll nearly always find trans fats hiding in our shopping trolleys in foods like margarine, sauces, commercially baked goods and snack foods like crackers. Food establishments are also fond of frying in partially hydrogenated oils. Of course they are! Tellingly, these fats are banned in Denmark and New York state because of the health risks they impose. Think grievous bodily harm in the nutritional courts.

Professor Walter Willet, Harvard School of Public Health, regards trans fats as 'the worst food-processing disaster in U.S. history'. Willet ascribes 100,000 unnecessary

American deaths each year to heart disease and the unregulated consumption of these noxious fats. While the FDA has called for compulsory labelling of trans fats on product packaging, foods with less than 0.5% apparently do not need to list it. Research shows, however, that even half a gram can have adverse effects on health. Canada set a different standard of 'zero' as being less than 0.2 grams. Not worried? We should be. Heart disease is Ireland's biggest killer, even bigger than cancer.

The good news? There are lots of heroic, unadulterated fats to play with in your kitchen. And they are crazy delicious. Look for unrefined extra virgin oils extracted from olives, avocados, nuts or seeds. These are your reliable friends. All are Mother Nature's favourite fats and have been shown to help raise the 'good' HDL cholesterol in our system as well as nourish proper liver function with their altruistic antioxidants. Given their megawatt health benefits, we should probably samba with these fats a little more. Let me help you do exactly that.

EXTRA VIRGIN COLD PRESSED COCONUT OIL ---------------------

All saturated fats are not equal. Each saturated fat has its own structure, and their individual differences influence the way they work in your body. (Scientists, look away while I mutilate your language.) Several saturated fats, called medium-chain triglycerides (MCTs), are metabolised more like carbohydrates than fats and are quickly used for energy. Coconut oil seems to be the best example, favoured by sporting icons like Gordon D'Arcy and Brendan Brazier. Pure palm oil is another, but it's tricky to find in its purest, unadulterated form. This is because pure palm oil is bright red and alarmingly whiffy. Commercial brands prefer to deodorise and bleach this beautiful red oil to make it more palatable, but it disfigures palm oil's health benefits.

Expect to get about 8g of MCT in 1 tablespoon of extra virgin coconut oil. Butter will deliver 1-2g and ghee around 4g. Bulletproof coffee relies on a distinctive MCT oil that is pure diesel for our mitochondria at 14g per tablespoon. This helps explain its energy-enhancing reputation, turning colleagues into amateur Tasmanian devils. MCT oil is, of course, created in a lab with isolated extracts of coconut and palm oils, so it hasn't won a place in my Hall of Fame. Nevertheless I'm interested in MCT oil's cult following and the impossibly delicious athletes thriving on it!

Coconut oil's real deal lies with its fancy immune-boosting compounds like lauric and caprylic acid. The predominant

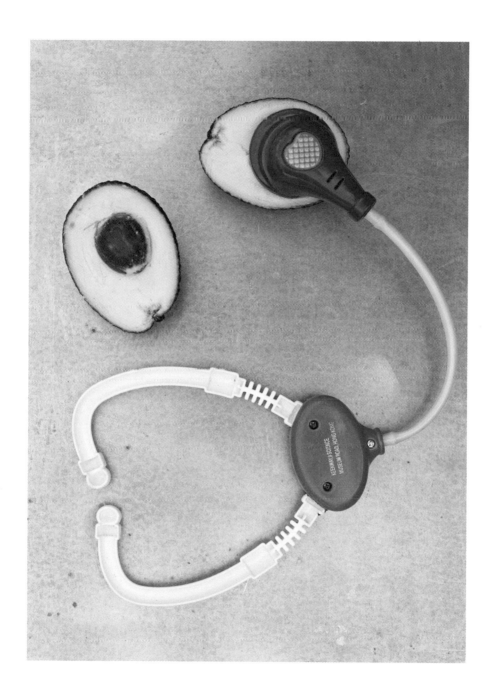

MCT in coconut oil seems to be lauric acid, known for its mega antimicrobial, antiviral and antibacterial properties. Think Ninjago in a tub. Much of the research on lauric and caprylic acids (also found in breast milk) has shown that certain pathogens can be deactivated by these MCTs.

EXTRA VIRGIN OLIVE OIL ------------------------------------

Extra virgin olive oil has been shown to help raise the 'good' HDL cholesterol in our system and lower the 'bad' LDL level, cheering up your overall cholesterol score. Olives have also been found to house jazzy health-enhancing compounds that are venerated in health circles. The first, oleocanthal, has fierce anti-inflammatory properties to help alleviate symptoms of high blood pressure. The second includes a range of active polyphenols that help to reduce blood pressure and the associated risk of coronary disease.

Please don't fry with extra virgin olive oil though, and try to make sure your oil is of the supertastic cold-pressed variety. Frying disfigures the oil's benefits, as the fatty acids start to decompose under high heat. Gentle sweating is okay though. It's probably worth looking for certified organic varieties to avoid the adulterated olive oils on the market.

GHEE ---

Okay, the name is unfortunate, but the ancients in Ayurvedic teachings (them ones with sagacity and sexperience) considered ghee to be the most sacred of foods because it enabled the 'goodness' from our diet to be absorbed. Scientists can now tell us why. Ghee, a sister of butter, is rich in fat-soluble vitamins A and D, without which some nutrients like calcium can't be synthesised in the body. Interesting, eh?

Yes, ghee is still saturated fat, but that doesn't bother me. What interests me most is this fat's nutritional whistle and its stability when heated in a frying pan. As soon as any fat reaches its smoke point (the point at which the fat begins to decompose and make free radicals), the fat will lose any nutritional purchase it once had. Free radicals are those nasty carcinogenic compounds that act like evil Power Rangers in your system. Not the sort of thing you want to serve your family.

Extra virgin olive oil has a smoke point of 180°C, so anything higher will disfigure the fat and mutilate its nutritional profile. Similarly, hemp oil has a low smoke point of 160°C and will foxtrot with your arteries if heated

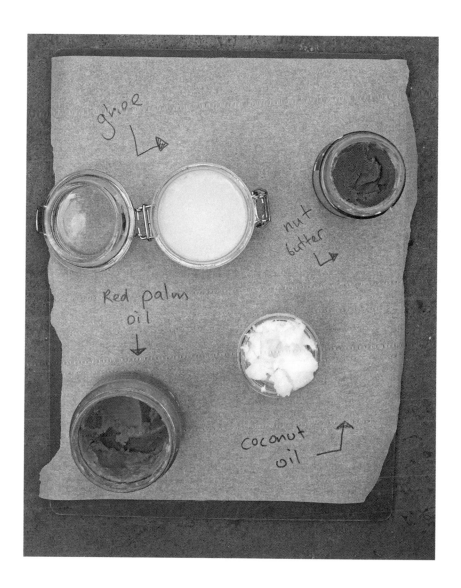

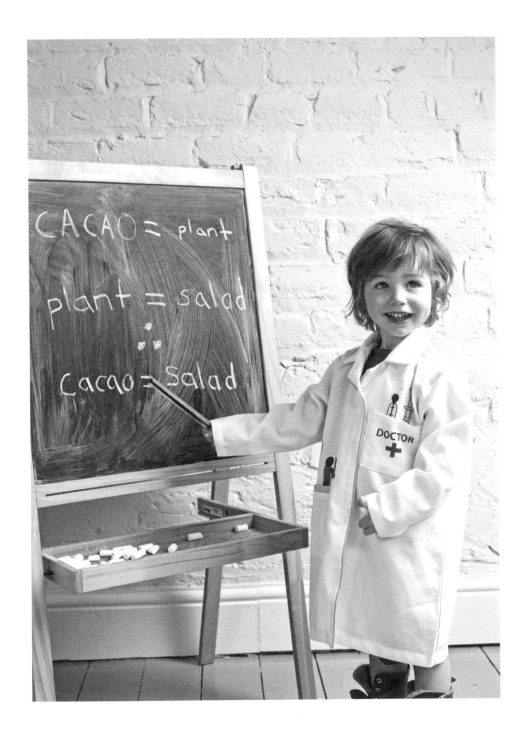

any higher. Hemp oil is awesome for salad dressings, so keep it away from the pan.

What do I use? Coconut oil, with a boastful smoke point of 220°C. But ghee is sneaking into Irish kitchens, without the threat of yogi pantaloons or Ayurvedic lentils. It has a similarly high smoke point of around 220°C.

Why not just use butter? I hear you! The milk solids (proteins and natural sugars) bring butter's smoke point down to 150°C. In the process of making ghee, these milk solids, including lactose, are removed, leaving only liquid gold and a house smelling of freshly baked shortbread. This markedly raises its smoke point. Nice one.

People who are diagnosed as lactose sensitive can often tolerate ghee, so it's worth trying. Making ghee is quicker than boiling pasta. You can find a recipe on my website, www.susanjanewhite.com. Gheelicious.

NUT AND SEED BUTTERS --

Plant-based butters are made by gently grinding nuts or seeds to release their naturally salubrious oils. They are amazing hives of nutrition and are gorgeous spread on bread and crackers. I feed my boys pumpkin seed sandwiches to boost their frontline defences every autumn. Pumpkin seeds are a good source of the immune-loving mineral zinc. This mineral is also responsible for proper hormone production and for healing bruised tissue.

Each nut or seed has its own unique health benefit. It's absolutely worth navigating them all! Most schools have a nut-free policy, so I think seed butters are the way forward.

SUNFLOWER OIL --

More often than not, commercial sunflower oil is a highly processed, nutritionally bankrupt product. I don't use it.

UNBLEACHED RED PALM OIL -------------------------------------

This stuff stinks. But for good reason. Extra virgin red palm oil contains blushing amounts of carotenoids - gram for gram, it has more than tomatoes and carrots. Carotenoids are precursors to vitamin A, that powerful antioxidant and immune charger.

Be sure to dodge the refined, bleached and deodorised varieties that are nutritionally worthless and are a favourite among food manufacturers. In its natural, untreated state, palm oil should be luminous red in colour from its high concentration of carotenes and tocols. It's not ideal for raw food dishes because of its honk. I use extra virgin palm oil at low temperatures to sweat vegetables intended for curries, which mask its strong taste. It's also mighty as a leg moisturiser in the summer if you don't mind the queer whiff.

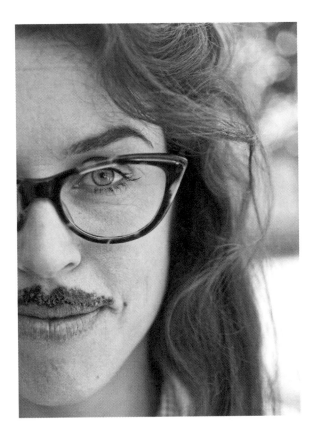

See Hot Cocoa recipe on p.70.

WHAT ABOUT WHEAT? AND GLUTEN?

If Ebola doesn't get us, gluten will.

Just kidding.

GSOH folks! Gluten is not a poison - let's get that straight. Gluten is not unhealthy either. For most people, gluten (a protein found in wheat, rye and barley) is more than tolerable, it's bleedin' great. Gluten is what makes baguettes fluffy and donuts spongy. So what's the problem?

It is estimated that one in 100 people cannot break down gluten. This is coeliac disease, an inflammatory condition where gluten irritates the digestive tract and can cause serious discomfort. Ireland has an impressive headcount of coeliacs, so we can't all blame Gwynnie.

The reality, however, might be a little more complicated because more than one in 100 are claiming to be gluten sensitive and are experiencing similar digestive discomfort. **There are many theories but no clear, scientifically satisfying answers**. Many respond well to FODMAP diets, an acronym for a series of carbohydrates that no one will ever remember: fermentable oligosaccharides, disaccharides, monosaccharides and polyols. For more on that, take a look at Professor Peter Gibson's research at Monash University.

Dr David Perlmutter, the godfather of glutards, is a popular neurologist whose research purports to link gluten and grains to Alzheimer's disease and depression. Controversial? I certainly think so. Grains aren't the problem - in fact, they're part of the solution to a healthy, varied diet. Our modern processed diet has bastardised grains, chiefly wheat, into a nutritionally void substance that most of us consume several times a day. Nearly one-third of the foods found on our supermarket shelves contain some component of nutritionally stripped wheat - usually gluten, starch or both. **It seems to me that wheat has turned into a bland industrial commodity**. The physical distress some people experience after eating commercial bread, for example, has less to do with grains or gluten than with the way large commercial bakeries operate. Instead of spending 48 hours making traditional bread, loaves are belched out on conveyor belts within a few minutes, designed to last for weeks on supermarket shelves. Commercial white flour in the US is often bleached using chemicals like acetone peroxide, chlorine and benzoyl peroxide. This is not real *bread*! Is it any wonder our bodies reject this stuff, manifesting its contempt for such foods through symptoms like constipation, bloating and gas? Your body is trying to talk to you. These symptoms are its language.

So what about spelt? The problem with heritage wheat like spelt, einkorn and dozens of others is that they don't produce a high yield. From an agronomic perspective, it's too risky for farmers to consider growing heirloom wheat varieties (unless they're loaded like Prince Charles and in the market for a new hobby). This leaves us with a standardised, highly processed variety in America, Ireland and the UK. There is a promising movement of scientists and adventurous bakers who are trying to resurrect older wheat grains. Emmer, faro, einkorn and kamut are all examples of gorgeous heritage wheat grains that taste far superior to the 'wheat' that you and I are accustomed to.

So if you're a member of the GF brigade or just giving wheat a break, count yourself lucky. There are stacks of groovy grains and flours to play with that may have otherwise never muscled for attention - quinoa, lentils, chickpeas, teff. These are your new badass friends. Many taste even better than regular wheat. Rosemary, olive and flaxseed bread instead of boring sliced pan. Mexican chilli beans, avocado and corn tacos in place of soggy pasta evenings. Still with me? **Sounds odd, but instead of feeling restricted by your food choices, expect to feel entirely liberated**.

Given that we are obsessed with wheat (cereals, bread, pasta, cake, biscuits, even sauces), it does make sense to diversify. Worst-case scenario? Your taste buds will flirt with new flavours and your mother-in-law will be engrossed by your brilliance.

The definition of insanity is doing the same thing over and over and expecting different results. Maybe it's time to make friends with these flours.

ALMOND FLOUR AND GROUND ALMONDS ----------------------------

We already know that nuts are spectacularly healthy and tasty, but the almond is the angel of the firmament. These perfumed nuts deserve wings of their own. Steaming with waist-friendly fats, age-defying vitamin E, bodybuilding protein and buff levels of calcium, what's not to love? Definitely my favourite sub for white flour.

BROWN RICE FLOUR --

This is the easiest gluten-free flour to start with, and the most obedient to use. It's practically ablaze with B

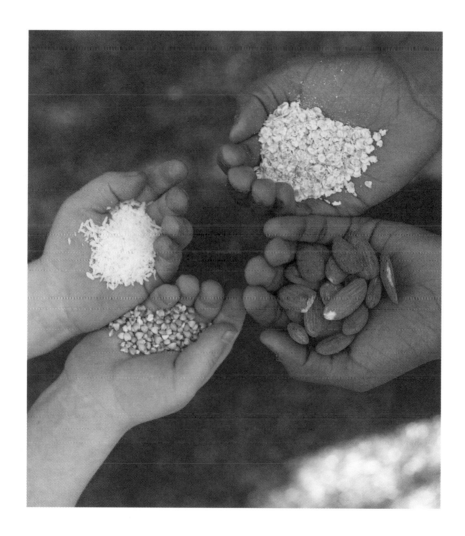

vitamins, which act like spark plugs in the body (especially important for indolent cabinet ministers). I like to pair it with my vegan buttermilk recipe to give it structure (see the Boozy Cherry Cupcakes on page 88). This helps bypass the inevitable crumbling mess that gluten-free baking can precipitate – stuff of nightmares for coeliacs.

BUCKWHEAT FLOUR --

Buckwheat is a small triangular grain confused by shades of red, brown and green. Japanese soba noodles, French galettes and Russian blini are made from buckwheat, so chances are you've already made friends with this wholegrain. Despite its name, buckwheat is not wheat. Hollywood's glitterati love this gluten-free carb because of its slow-release energy and beautifying bioflavonoids. Buckwheat even has lysine, that elusive amino acid that helps prevent outbreaks of pesky cold sores. Like many of these flours, buckwheat is loaded with battery-boosting B vitamins. Think B for brain, B for buckwheat.

CHESTNUT FLOUR --

Chestnut flour is naturally sweet and rich in fibre. Italians have been using chestnut flour for centuries, y'all. These folks seem to know a lot about tickling taste buds. If you have some vegan guests for Christmas this year, they'll go ballistic for the Boozy Cherry Cupcakes on page 88 that incorporate chestnut flour. Health geeks have lovebombed this flour of late, so supplies could be hard to find. Best make friends with your local stockist or an unsuspecting Italian.

CHICKPEA FLOUR, BESAN FLOUR, GRAM FLOUR --------------------

There's a good reason they're not called bloke peas: chickpeas are puffed with feline-friendly compounds. There's magnesium, a mineral many of us crave once a month when we become a crazed version of a slightly less bonkers self. Magnesium has the magnificent ability to relieve cramps by helping our blood vessels relax. Good news for headaches and varicose veins too.

Then there's isoflavones, a plant-based phyto-oestrogen considered useful in the fight against breast cancer. It looks like our body converts isoflavones into compounds that mimic some of the effects of oestrogen. Why is this important? Because the female reproductive system is influenced by oestrogen. Studies on the specific benefits of plant-based phyto-oestrogens have yielded mixed results, but they seem to have some correlation to a reduced risk of hormonal cancers and may even play a role in bone density. (Personally, I think my Pilates instructor plays a bigger role in bone density than any conceivable food. He's so hot no one ever misses a class.) Phyto-oestrogens have already been used to improve menopausal symptoms. Some women prefer to take phyto-oestrogens rather than opt for hormone replacement therapy (HRT). I do like the idea of being prescribed hummus for hot flushes!

COCONUT FLOUR --

Coconut flour is quite the diva. It's the Gordon Ramsay of flours. You can't substitute it with any other flour. Try to, and your baked goodies will throw a hissy in the oven. This is because coconut flour demands alarming quantities of liquid in comparison to plain white flour.

I'm prepared to put up with coconut flour's shenanigans because it makes a really great alternative to gluten or grain flours (hello paleo, hello coeliac). You won't beat this flour's fibre content either, ringing in at a whopping 42% (bye bye, haemorrhoids).

MILLED FLAXSEED (LINSEED) AND MILLED CHIA SEED -------------

Chia and flax provide snazzy essential fats to get your frontal lobe raving. Red Bull for the brain.

It's worth noting that the type of omega-3 fatty acid found in flax and chia is slightly different than those found in oily fish. Flax and chia contain ALA, the precursor to EPA and DHA fatty acids. You've probably come across these confusing terms at the pharmacy when choosing omega-3 supplements. In short, EPA and DHA are easier for the body to assimilate. Therefore, you'll find stronger doses of omega-3 in oily fish, but you won't find cancer-protecting lignans and cholesterol-lowering plant sterols, both of which the flax and chia seed can gloat about. There's a surprising amount of calcium wrangled in there too. 'Tis a fine food.

Milled flax and chia can also be used to replace eggs in baking. Mix 1 tablespoon of either with 3 tablespoons of water or some other liquid. Magic.

OATS ---

The soluble fibre in oats, beta-glucan, gives this carb its superstar status. Beta-glucans are a chain of immune-boosting polysaccharides, similar to those found in medicinal mushrooms. But they've also been shown to benefit heart health by latching onto cholesterol in the bowels and banishing it like unwanted vermin.

The other type of fibre, insoluble fibre, has the ability to police our bowels, improving congestion and reducing transit time like a tenacious traffic warden. Oats and dried fruit contain astral amounts of the stuff.

Oats have additional gloating cards. B vitamins will recharge spent batteries and frayed nerves, while their slow-release carbs will have our toes cha-cha-ing all day long. Oats are naturally gluten free but are often processed in the same industrial plants as wheat, barley and rye, resulting in cross-contamination. If you aren't coeliac, then this won't affect you. Oats contain a protein called avenin, initially thought to be similar to gluten. According to Coeliac UK, most coeliacs can happily tolerate avenin and do not present with avenin antibodies. If you're worried, ask your GP or dietician for more advice.

This grain is a nutritional darling. I promise it's much easier to bake with than pronounce.

Quinoa (*keen-wah*) is a mighty South American staple that looks like couscous, only tastes better. Unusually for a carb, quinoa contains all the essential amino acids required to make a 'complete' source of protein. That's a high-five for bench pressers and vegetarians. Just one cup of cooked quinoa will gift you with 10g of protein and a honking 16mg of chest-thumping iron. Little wonder the Incan army marched on it (erm, metaphorically, not literally).

In 2014, quinoa was trendier than Wes Anderson. Rumours of Western markets stealing Peru's indigenous food from its own people spread like Chinese whispers and tormented many a vegan's soul. According to the United Nations, the opposite is closer to the truth. Our markets have supported the expansion of quinoa farms across tricky non-arable land. The sort of terrain that quinoa, and little else, thrives on. So now you know why Alicia Silverstone sleeps soundly at night.

Sorghum is a type of millet, with nearly twice as much iron. Phwoar. It's particularly high in fibre too and is naturally sweeter than the average grain. I use Bob's Red Mill 'Sweet' Sorghum Flour but always combine it with psyllium husks to help achieve a fluffy consistency in baked goods.

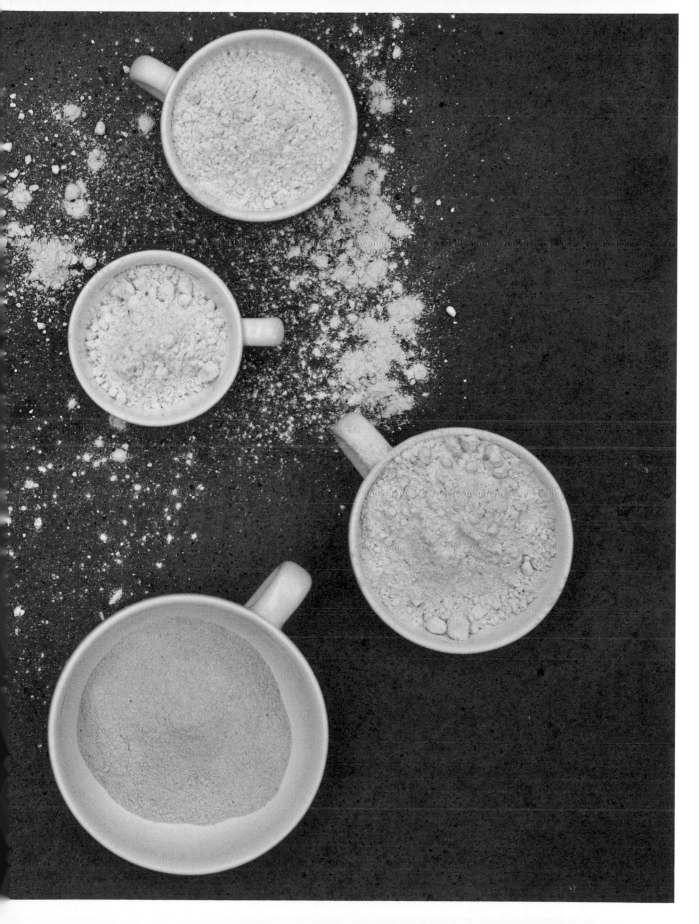

I don't altogether like the taste of millet, so I use it as a vehicle for flavour. It makes alarmingly good donuts (page 146) and muffins (page 86). Sorghum is gluten free.

TEFF FLOUR --

It's here. The latest superfood, all the way from Ethiopia. (Calm down. Teff is produced in Idaho too, where most of our supplies originate. Don't go tweeting Geldof.)

Teff is a whole grain that boasts similar nutritional strengths as quinoa and amaranth, although it's noticeably smaller: a single grain of teff measures less than 1mm in diameter. Think of it as mutant quinoa, ranging from black to red and from ivory to brown. But teff has a mild flavour and is naturally sweet. Move over, quinoa. Your fifteen minutes are up.

If you suffer from volcanic cold sores, teff will help ramp up your system with banks of lysine. This is an important amino acid responsible for confusing the herpes virus and preventing or lessening outbreaks of cold sores. When that tingling sensation arrests your bottom lip, it's also useful to steer clear of foods rich in arginine (the virus's preferred fodder). Arginine-rich foods include peanuts, red meat and spinach. Oh well.

TIPS FROM A TART

There's little point horsing into healthy food unless it tastes good. Life is too short to tax your taste buds, don't you think?

NEW TO ALL THIS? ----------

Pomegranate Halva (page 162)
Raspberry Jam - The Healthy Kind (page 133)
American Peanut Butter Cookies (page 137)

TIRED? ----------------------

Matcho Latte (page 63)
Hot Shots (page 77)
Spirulina Grenades (page 186)

BUSY? ----------------------

Mega Raspberry Bombs (page 182)
Chocolate Seed Soldiers (page 158)
Brainiac Brownies (page 93)

PMT? ------------------------

Health by Chocolate (page 190)
Earl Grey Chocolate Tartlets (page 101)
BBQ Kale Crisps (page 126)

FABULOUS BREAKFASTS? -------

Apple and Winter Squash Crumble (page 150)
Birch Sugar Granola (page 171) with Coconut Milk Yoghurt (page 130)
Hipsteria (page 68)
MILF Muffins (page 86)
Chia Breakfast Pud with Passion Fruit and Sea Salt (page 149)

RUBBISH AT THE OFFICE? -----

Toasted Pecans (page 174)
Teff, Ginger and Black Pepper Cookies (page 134)
Peppermint-Laced Energy Balls (page 189)
Secret Agent Gingerbread (page 155)
Probiotic Coffee (page 83)

MOST POPULAR RECIPES? ------

Pomegranate Halva (page 162)
Chocolate Seed Soldiers (page 158)
Lemon Shizzle Cake (page 115)
Brainiac Brownies (page 93)
Banoffee Mess (page 98)

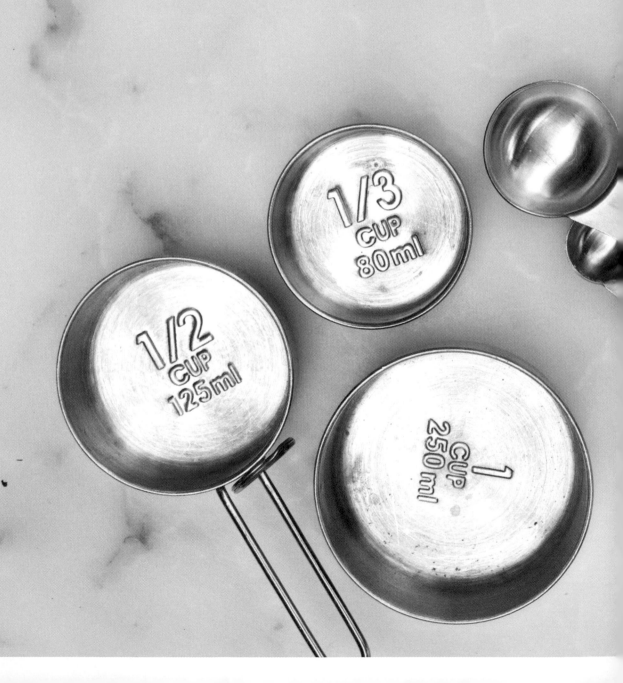

A NOTE ON
THE MEASUREMENTS
USED IN THIS BOOK

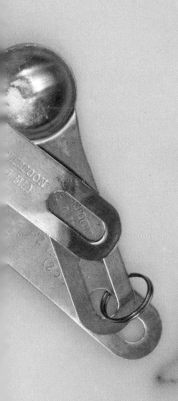

1 British/Australian cup = 250ml

1/4 cup = 60ml

1/3 cup = 80ml

1/2 cup = 125ml

2/3 cup = 165ml

3/4 cup = 190ml

1 tablespoon = 15ml

Why do I use cups? I think cups are friendlier and make it easier to visualise quantities while jotting down your shopping list. The metric system can alienate people in the kitchen. It has a disempowering effect. Do you know what 65 grams of almonds look like? Or 325 grams of rye? Me neither. But don't worry, I've included both cups and grams throughout the book to suit all camps. I just thought it was worth explaining my crazy-lady vibe.

1

VIRGIN DRINKS

YOUR INNER HEALTH BITCH

HAZELNUT MILK

****

I call these 'grandpa nuts' because they're wonderfully nourishing for seniors. Here's why: hazelnuts contain beta-sitosterol, a groovy compound shown to help benign prostatic hyperplasia. That's doctor speak for the numerous trips men over 60 take to the loo during the night. While benign prostatic hyperplasia isn't harmful, it can be a darned nuisance.

A study in The Lancet revealed that patients given 20mg of beta-sitosterol three times a day demonstrated a reduction in those midnight dashes. Okay, so this is significantly more beta-sitosterol than one hazelnut can provide, but nevertheless, it's one of many sources that can be easily included in Grandpa's diet. And no, Nutella doesn't count. Nice try.

$^3/_4$ cup (110g) raw hazelnuts
$^1/_4$ cup (35g) raw almonds
1–2 Medjool dates, stones
  removed
3 cups (750ml) filtered water
1 nut milk bag or muslin
  cloth

Makes 3 cups (750ml)

Put your hazelnuts and almonds in a large bowl, cover with cold filtered water and soak them overnight.

In the morning, rinse and drain the soaked nuts. Tumble into a blender along with the pitted dates and 3 cups (750ml) filtered water. Pelt on the highest setting for 20 seconds.

Wash your hands thoroughly before the next step to avoid spoiling the milk. Place a nut milk bag into a large bowl and slowly pour the nut milk and pulp into the bag. Gently twist the top of the bag and use your hands to squeeze the milk into the bowl, which should take about 20 seconds. My children love doing this.

Discard the dry pulp in the cloth and pour your milk into a scrupulously clean bottle with a screw-top lid. Add more water if it's too thick.

Nut milk will last in the fridge for up to three days. Give the jar a jolly good shake before enjoying or use it in recipes throughout the book.

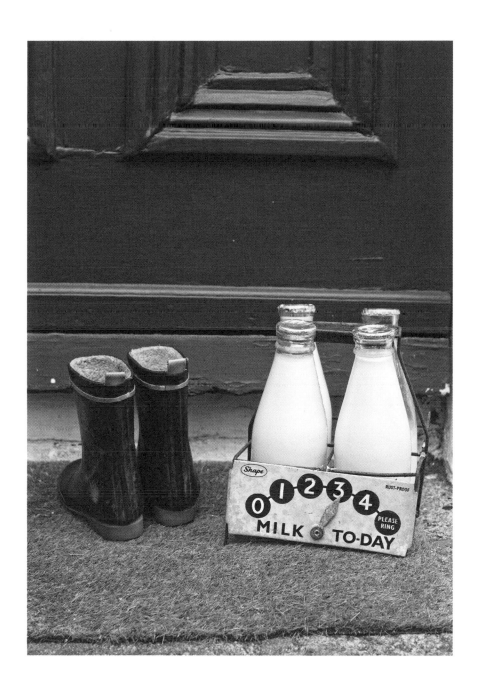

VIRGIN DRINKS

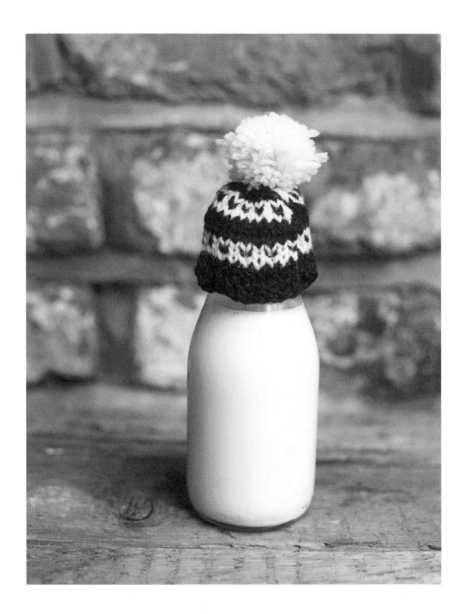

GOLDEN TURMERIC MILK

****

This spiced turmeric milk tastes like the most scrumptious vanilla ice cream, melted into a tall glass. Order it at Pressed Juicery in Los Angeles, a church for vegans and savvy celebs. For the rest of us, here is their hallowed recipe.

Place the almonds in a large bowl, cover with cold filtered water and soak them overnight or for 10-12 hours. Some health advocates advise soaking nuts in salted water, but food scientist Harold McGee observed that this was merely folklore and can in fact leach calcium and water-soluble vitamins from the food.

In the morning, rinse and drain the almonds. Add the soaked almonds to a powerful blender along with no more than 2 cups (500ml) of fresh filtered water and the remaining ingredients. Blend on super nasty high until foamy. A Vitamix, Nutribullet or OmniBlend will do this in 15 seconds. A regular blender will take about 60 seconds. Food processors are usually not strong enough to make nut milk.

Wash your hands thoroughly before the next step to avoid spoiling the milk. Place a nut milk bag or muslin cloth over a large bowl. Pour the contents of your blender into the cloth and strain it. A fabulous creamy milk will collect in the bowl underneath. Gently twist the top of the bag and use your hands to squeeze the milk into the bowl, which should take about 20 seconds. A deliciously cathartic job.

Discard the dry pulp in the cloth and pour your golden turmeric milk into a scrupulously clean bottle with a screw-top lid. It will last in the fridge for up to three days.

A toast, to eternity!

1 cup (140g) raw almonds
2 cups (500ml) filtered water
chunk of fresh ginger, unpeeled
1 tablespoon raw local honey
1 teaspoon ground turmeric or a good chunk of fresh turmeric
1 teaspoon ground cinnamon
2 green cardamom pods
1 nut milk bag or muslin cloth

Makes 2 cups (500ml)

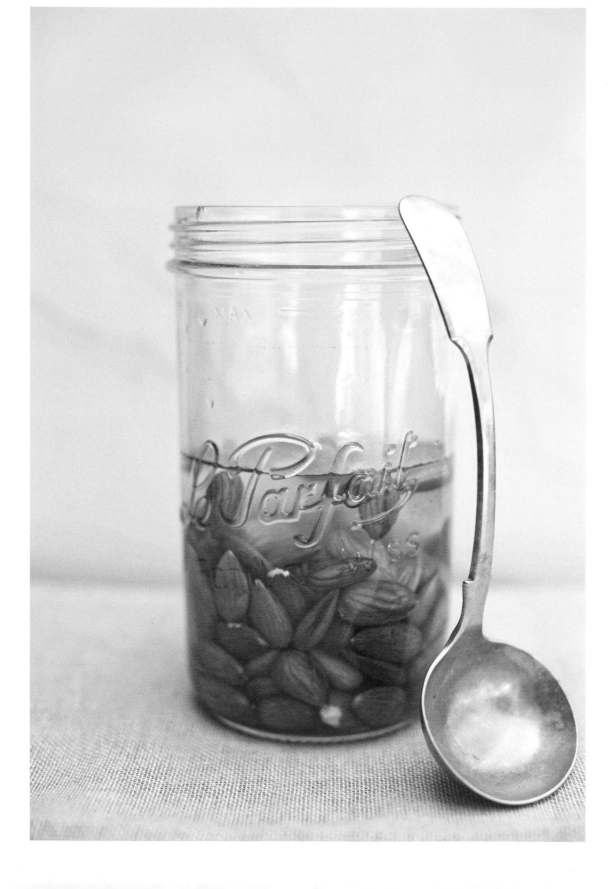

ALMOND AND HEMP MILK

****

We already know that nuts are incredibly virtuous and tasty, but the almond is the angel of the firmament. These perfumed nuts deserve wings of their own. Try to source organic almonds, most of which escape gassing. Non-organic almonds are regularly subjected to this controversial process in order to preserve them for longer.

When soaked, almonds are considered to be alkaline as opposed to acidic. Why is this important? Because acidic foods are thought to make calcium absorption more difficult in the body. A yogi's worst nightmare. Actually, scrap that. An accidental bottom burp during downward facing dog on a yoga mat beside Colin Farrell is way worse. So I hear.

Alkaline foods, such as fresh fruit and vegetables, help our bones access and utilise the calcium from our diet more efficiently. This doesn't mean acidic foods are unhealthy, but suggests that balancing acid with alkaline is important for strong bones. And supple dance floor moves. The alkaline-acid theory always sounded a little hocus pocus until I researched calcium retention after popping out my two brutes. Luckily, alkaline foods are fabulously tasty so it's not a big ask to bulk up on them.

Brendan Brazier, a professional Ironman athlete, relies solely on a plant-based diet to fuel his training sessions (and his egg-box abs). I notice almonds get some serious adulation in his cookbook. Loaded with waist-friendly fats, body-building protein and age-defying minerals, these everyday nuts have been neglected in my life for far too long. And perhaps my body shows as much. I hereby resolve to eat more of them if it brings me closer to badass Brendan. And given my stats, plant-based calcium is something I'm on high alert for these days. All the better if I'm inspired by hot Californian athletes.

1 cup (140g) raw almonds
4 tablespoons shelled hemp
  seeds
3 cups (750ml) filtered water
2 Medjool dates, stones
  removed, or a splash of
  raw honey
$^1/_2$ vanilla pod or $^1/_2$
  teaspoon vanilla extract
  (optional)
1 nut milk bag

Makes 3-4 cups (750ml-
1 litre)

Place the almonds and hemp seeds in a large bowl, cover with cold filtered water and soak them overnight or for 10-12 hours. Some health enthusiasts insist on adding salt, but according to the world's greatest food scientist, Harold McGee, this is not only unnecessary but can leach important minerals. I'm with the dude in the white coat.

In the morning, rinse and drain. Clock them into your blender or Vitamix with 3 cups (750ml) filtered water, the dates and the snapped vanilla pod. Blend furiously for 15 seconds.

Wash your hands thoroughly before the next step to avoid spoiling the milk. Pour into a nut milk bag set inside a large bowl. Secure the top of the nut bag and use your fingers to squeeze all the liquid from the pulp. It's so much fun for kids.

Discard the dry pulp and pour the fabulous creamy hemp milk into a scrupulously clean bottle with a screw-top lid. Store in the fridge and drink within three days.

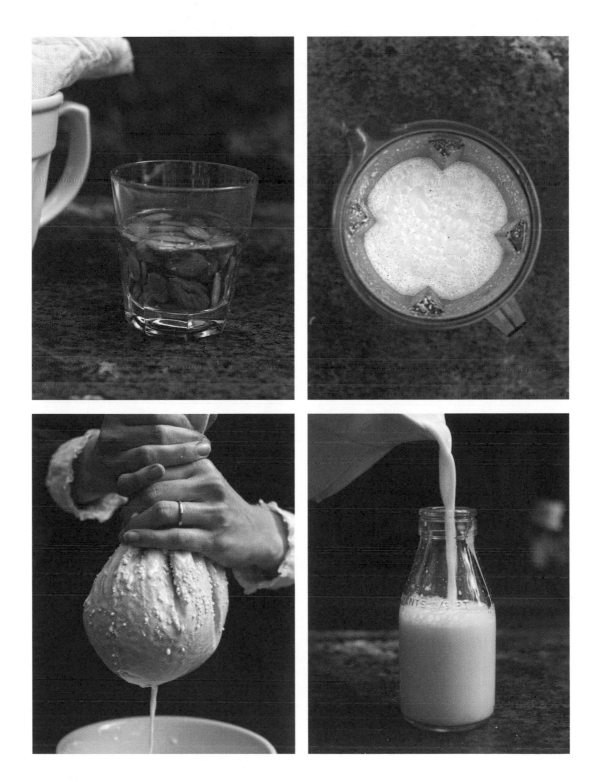

VIRGIN DRINKS

'WHOEVER SNUCK THE "S" IN FAST FOOD WAS A CLEVER LITTLE BASTARD.'

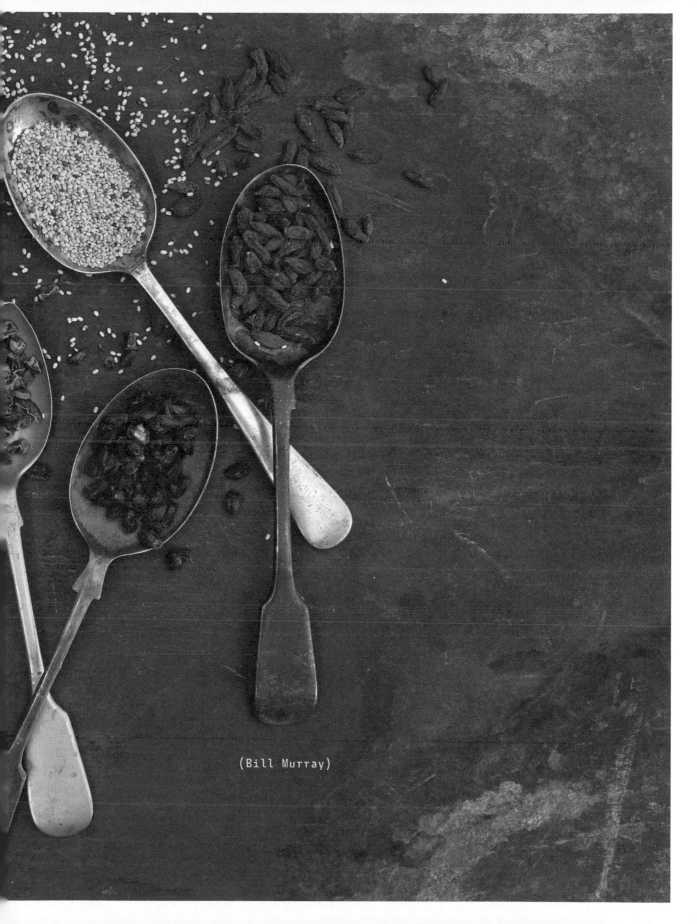

(Bill Murray)

BLACK SESAME MILK

****

Meet my biggest food crush: black sesame milk (and Katie Sanderson). Lord have mercy on us.

1 cup (140g) raw almonds or
  cashews
3-4 cups (750ml-1 litre)
  filtered water
1 teaspoon of your preferred
  sweetener
1 teaspoon extra virgin
  coconut oil (optional)
pinch of fine sea salt
4 tablespoons black sesame
  seeds

Makes 3 cups (750ml)

Soak the nuts in cold filtered water overnight. Cashews are much cheaper than almonds at the moment and work beautifully. Cashews only require 6 hours soaking too.

In the morning, drain and discard the soaking liquid and rinse the nuts under running water. Tumble the wet nuts into your blender (mine's an Omniblend, the poor man's Vitamix). Add the fresh filtered water, a touch of sweetener (I like using 1 Medjool date with the stone removed), the optional coconut oil and a pinch of sea salt.

At this stage you can just add the black sesame seeds, but Katie toasts them to bring out their extraordinary rhythm. Toss them onto a scorching hot, dry frying pan for 30 seconds. That's it. You can toast them on a dry baking tray in the oven too, but preheating the oven will take much longer.

Blend on high for 30 seconds or until the neighbours start shouting.

Wash your hands thoroughly before the next step to avoid spoiling the milk. Place a nut milk bag or muslin cloth over a bowl. Pour the contents of the blender into the cloth and strain it. A fabulous creamy milk will collect in the bowl underneath. You'll need to use your hands to squeeze everything through, not forgetting to secure the top by twisting the cloth or bag. Discard or compost the leftover dry pulp, as most of the nutrition has been transferred to the milk at this stage.

Pour your sesame milk into a pristinely clean bottle with a screw-top lid and refrigerate for up to three days. I pour it over granola and porridge and use it in baking, but it's also criminally good with coffee.

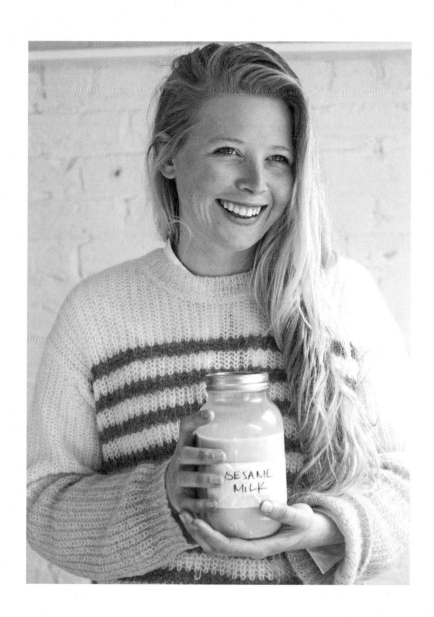

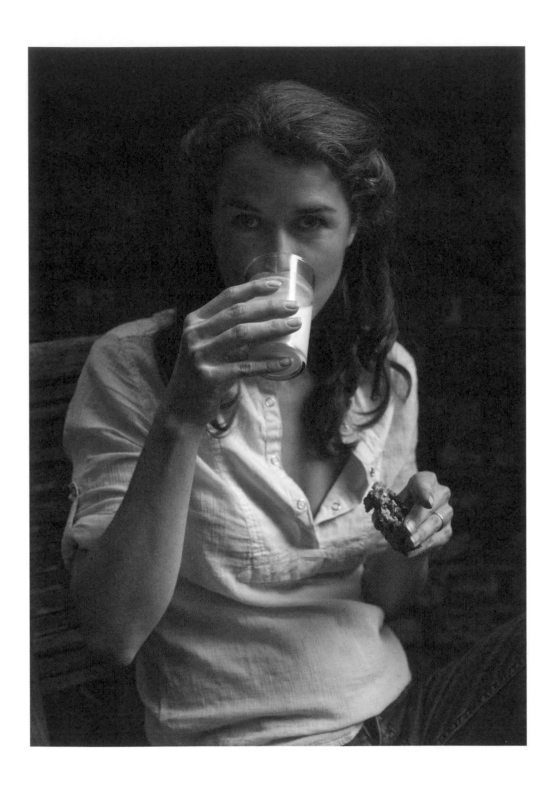

ALMOND MILK CHAI LATTE

****

Just when you thought you had dusted off the damage done by teenage years of Bros, Rick Astley and overexcited sebaceous glands, in creep wrinkles and saggy boobs. You'd think that if you suffered from the former, life would award you a pass on the latter. But science is rarely that beautiful.

Luckily, Mother N has a stash of ingredients in her medicine cabinet to help fight the ageing process. Almonds are buffed up with vitamin E, that special nutrient designed to tamper with ageing skin. It works by protecting fats from being mugged by free radicals. Scientists are in agreement that organisms age when cells accumulate free radical damage (stress, poor food choices, pollution). So I've turned to quaffing almond milk and feel more virtuous than a canonised nun.

Please don't guffaw at the fat content of almonds. These nuts are rich in monounsaturated fats, the ones your doc keeps begging you to eat. Monounsaturated fats are associated with reduced levels of cholesterol and a lower risk of heart disease, which is currently Ireland's number one killer. I love almonds' cargo of protein and calcium too. I feel a ballad coming on.

Boil the kettle and let your chai teabag steep in the hot water in a large mug covered with a plate for 8 minutes.

Meanwhile, gently warm the almond or other plant-based milk. Be sure not to let it boil. Remove the teabag and pour the milk over the spiced tea. Dust with cinnamon or maca and slurp away an evening with Netflix. For long summer evenings, slurp over ice.

1 sweet chai tea bag
1/4 cup (60ml) hot water
1 cup (250ml) plant-based
  milk (I use almond milk)
pinch of ground cinnamon or
  maca, to dust

Serves 1

CAFFEINE-FREE NIGHTCAP

****

My gran told me that roasted chicory was a coffee replacement during the war, but without the caffeine kick. So this is my caffeine-free, creamy hot drink before I hit the pillow. Beyond Bach.

1 cup (250ml) nut milk
2 teaspoons roasted chicory
  granules

Serves 1

I warm my milk with a Nespresso foamer and pour it over 2 teaspoons of roasted chicory granules, or you can heat the milk in a small saucepan and then whizz in a blender for some serious foam. Same same. Feel free to experiment with all sorts of plant-based milk and sweeten if necessary. Hazelnut or black sesame milk rock.

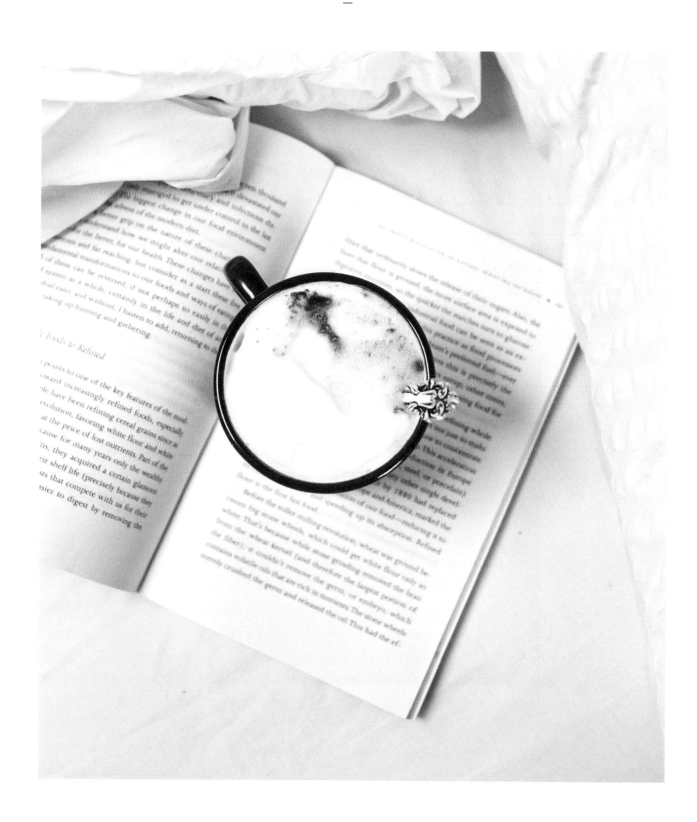

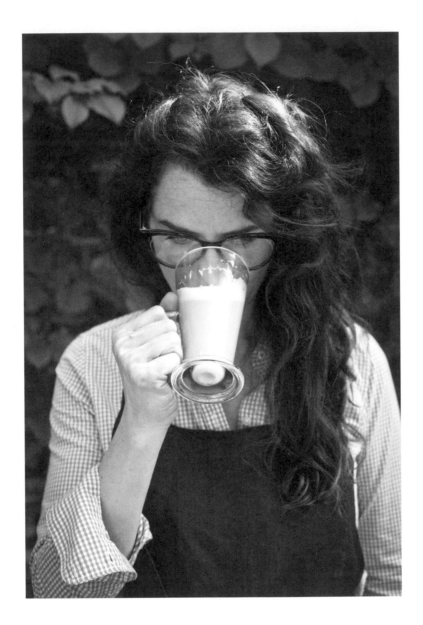

MATCHO LATTE

****

Matcha is the Katie Taylor of green teas: Olympian. Other green teas are still impressive, but matcha is high octane and inimitable.

Warm your preferred milk and honey in a small saucepan and add the matcha. Macadamia nut milk is The Shizzle. Whizz with a stick blender to help froth it up and serve immediately. If you have a Nespresso foamer, it will do everything for you while you sigh with adoration.

just under 1 cup (220ml)
  plant-based milk
honey to sweeten, if
  required
1/2 teaspoon matcha green tea
  powder

Serves 1

'FOOD IS NOT JUST CALORIES, IT IS INFORMATION. IT TALKS TO YOUR DNA AND TELLS IT WHAT TO DO.'

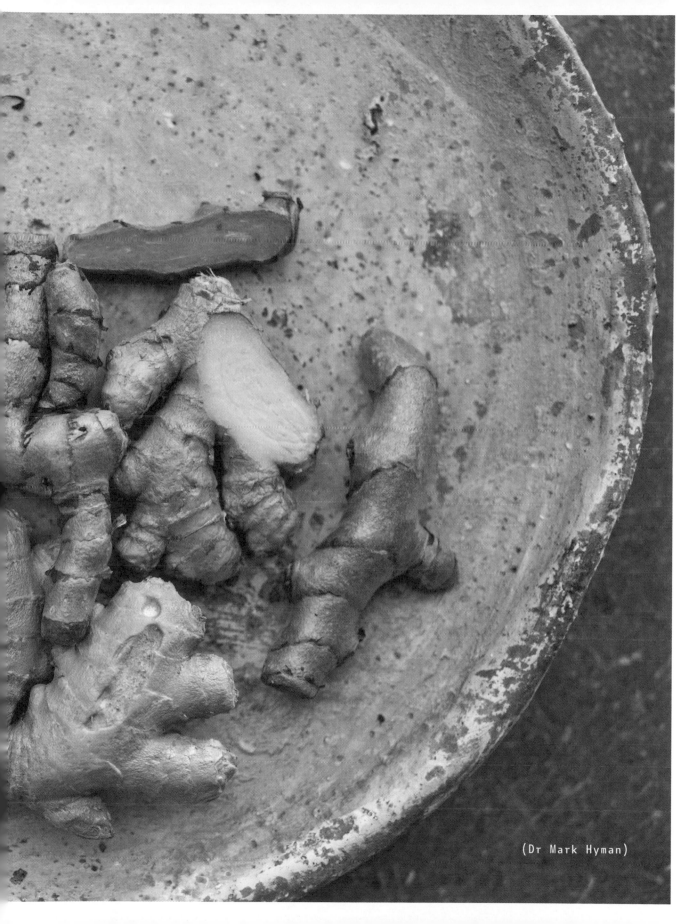
(Dr Mark Hyman)

COFFEE AND ALMOND MILKSHAKE

* *

This chilled bevy owns the summer like Miley Cyrus owns twerking - but more tasteful, I promise.

If coffee ain't your thang, bee pollen will get your veins doing the cha cha. It's an extraordinarily healthy food but it tastes like fermented dust balls, so I like to freeze all the flavour from it. If the queen bee thrives on it, sign me up! Unusually for a plant substance, bee pollen contains at least 18 amino acids, making it a whopping member of the protein clan. It's naturally rich in enzymes to stoke digestion and B vitamins to resuscitate dead batteries. Madame Queen needs to lay hundreds of eggs, daily, and lives 40 times longer than the worker bee, so her stamina is probably testament to this luminous superfood.

1/2 large banana, peeled and
  cut into discs
1 Medjool date, stone
  removed
shy of 1 cup (200ml)
  unsweetened almond milk
1 shot of espresso (or
  1 teaspoon frozen bee
  pollen)
1 tablespoon almond butter

Serves 1-3

Freeze the banana slices on a piece of parchment or non-stick paper. I tend to have a cargo of frozen banana discs at the ready to service tired friends and limbs. When the bananas are frozen solid, pitch them into a high-speed food processor alongside the remaining ingredients. If you can't find Medjool dates, you can replace them with pre-soaked regular dates and a prayer.

Blend on high. Pour into chilled jam jars and sip away the boredom at your bus stop.

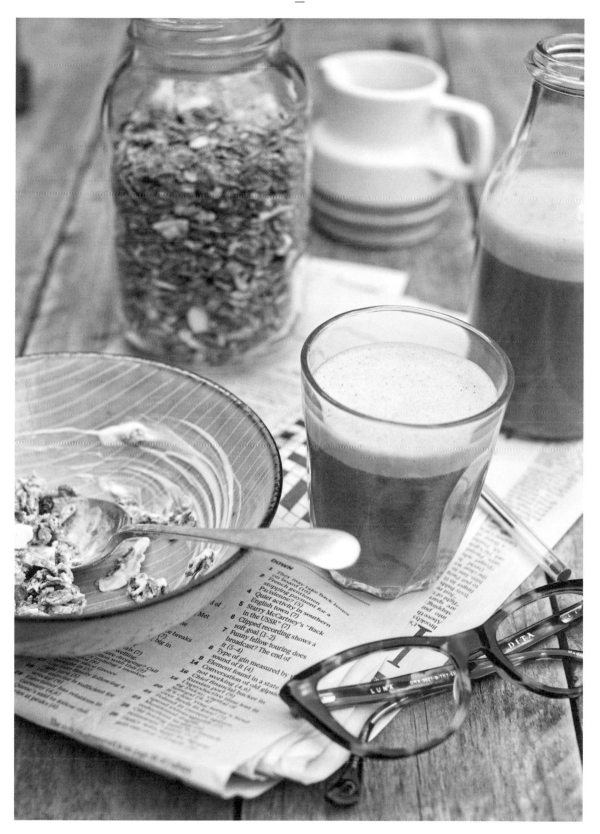

VIRGIN DRINKS

HIPSTERIA - PEANUT BUTTER CHOCOLATE SHAKE

* *

Raw cacao is the new kale. The difference between cacao and cocoa is simple. Cacao is raw, while cocoa is heat-treated. Both come from the same plant, and even the same pod. That's not to say one is good and the other is bad. Let me put it this way: Lisa Hannigan is the cacao of pop stars - raw, husky and unadulterated - to Rihanna's refined, cosmetic vibe. One is artisan and delicate; the other manufactured to excite every population on this planet. Which is more important? That's for you to decide.

1 banana, peeled and cut
  into discs
2-4 Medjool dates, stones
  removed
2 cups (500ml) plant-
  based milk (almond, oat,
  hazelnut)
2 tablespoons pure peanut
  butter
1 tablespoon raw cacao or
  cocoa powder

Serves 2-4

This is exceedingly good, so begin by blessing yourself. (I'm not religious and enjoy misplacing my reverence.) Freeze the banana slices on a piece of parchment or non-stick paper for a minimum of 40 minutes. Make sure the pieces aren't touching each other. Frozen banana is the ultimate trick for making creamy non-dairy smoothies, but you can replace it with half a ripe avocado if you're trying to cut down on sweetness.

Next, plug in a high-speed blender and add your dates, plant-based milk (I use almond milk), peanut butter and cacao powder. Whizz on full power until sumptuously smooth.

Serve in a tall glass and genuflect.

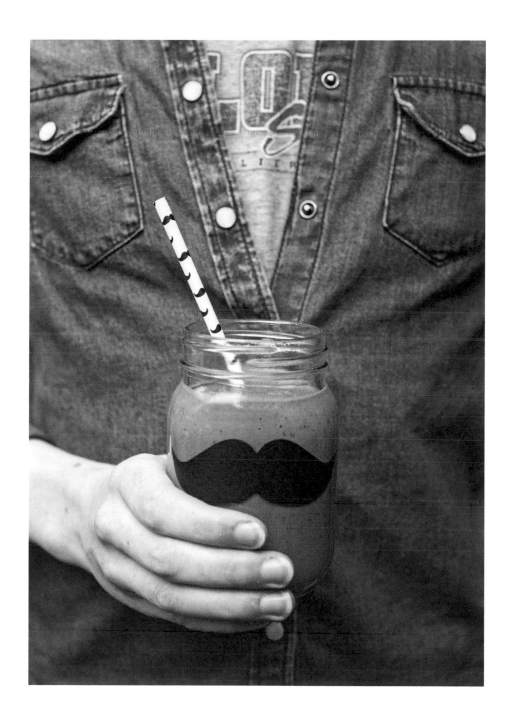

VIRGIN DRINKS

THE HOT COCOA

****

The cacao bean grows from a tree. And trees are plants. So chocolate is basically salad, right?

2 cups (500ml) unsweetened
plant-based milk
2 tablespoons cacao or cocoa
powder
2 tablespoons hazelnut
butter
1 tablespoon coconut sugar
or 2 teaspoons date syrup

Serves 2-6

Using a high-powered blender, whizz all the ingredients until foamy. Sounds like a pain in the arse, but it's the key step. Transfer to a mini saucepan and gently warm to your preferred temperature.

Run the blender jug under water to clean it, because if you forget, it's much harder to scrub later.

Pour into two mugs, four dainty cups or six espresso glasses. Kick back with your favourite friends and Fats Waller — or whatever makes your tail wag.

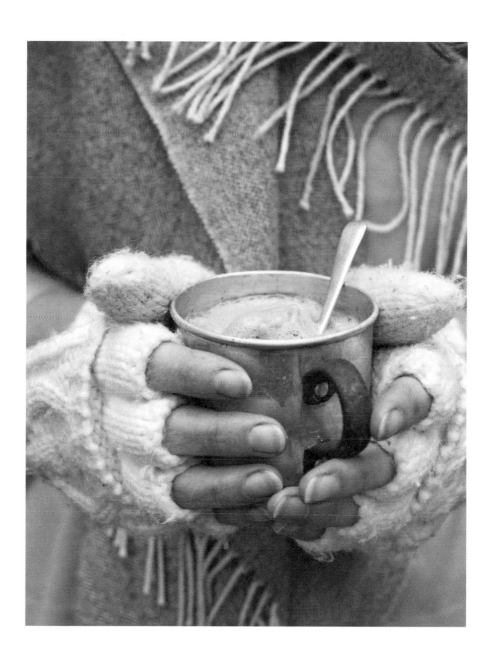

SMARTER PEOPLE PAY THE GROCER, NOT THE DOCTUR.

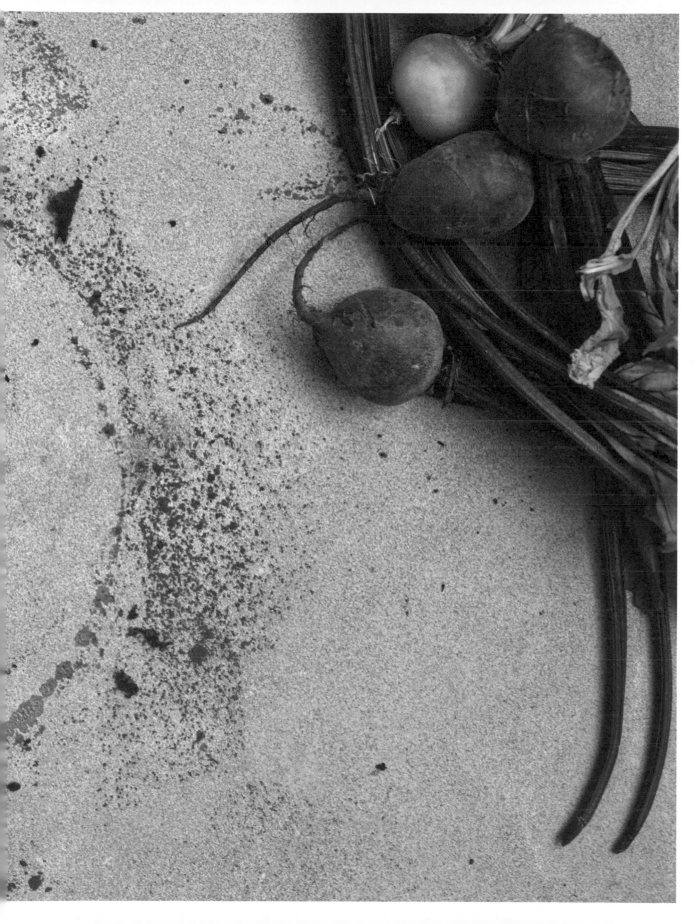

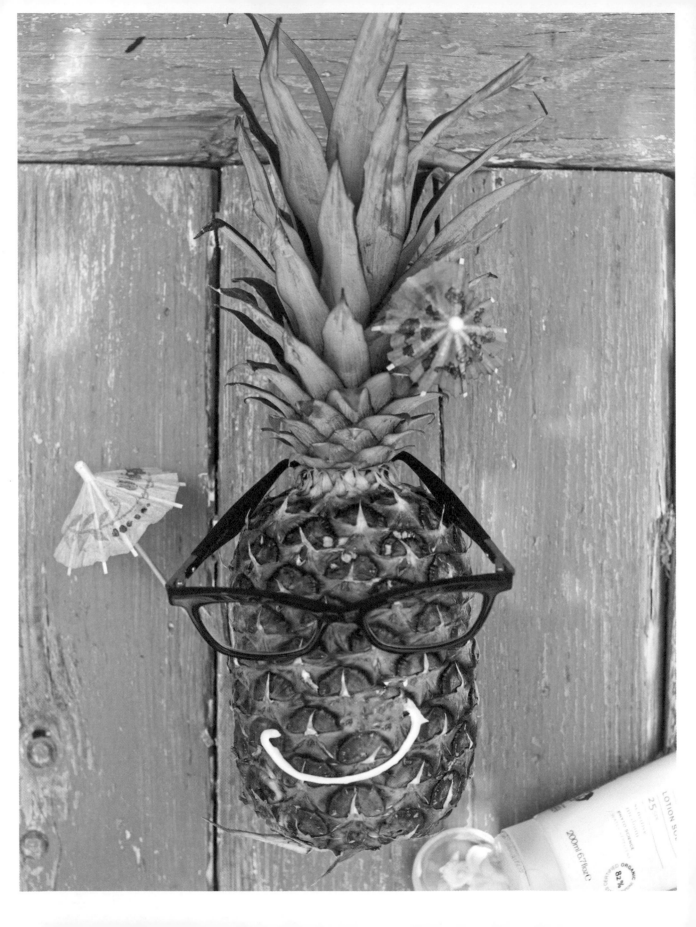

PIÑA KALEADA

****

Kale is an excellent source of folate, which is often associated with great-quality nookie. Looks like folate can regulate the production of histamine, a very important chemical released during orgasm. No, a cabbage smoothie will not bring you to climax, but you're welcome to try.

You probably don't need another reason to watch your folate intake, but here's an additional fireworks display you'll be interested in: folate plays a large role in our mental and emotional health. It is, in fact, a B vitamin – think B for brain and battery. Or Bergman and Bogart (okay, that's probably E for electricity, but you get the picture).

This mocktail is for those times when your body feels like a steaming Petri dish. The biggest surprise is that my children love it more than chocolate chip ice cream.

In a powerful blender, show these ingredients who's boss. Strain through a fine-mesh sieve and collect the rich nectar in a bowl set underneath it. Pour into pre-chilled glasses with lots of ice and dinky straws.

1 cup (250ml) coconut water
  or light coconut milk
2 slices of fresh pineapple,
  skin and
  core removed
2 stalks of kale, juiced
juice of 1 small lime
pinch of ground turmeric

Serves 2-4

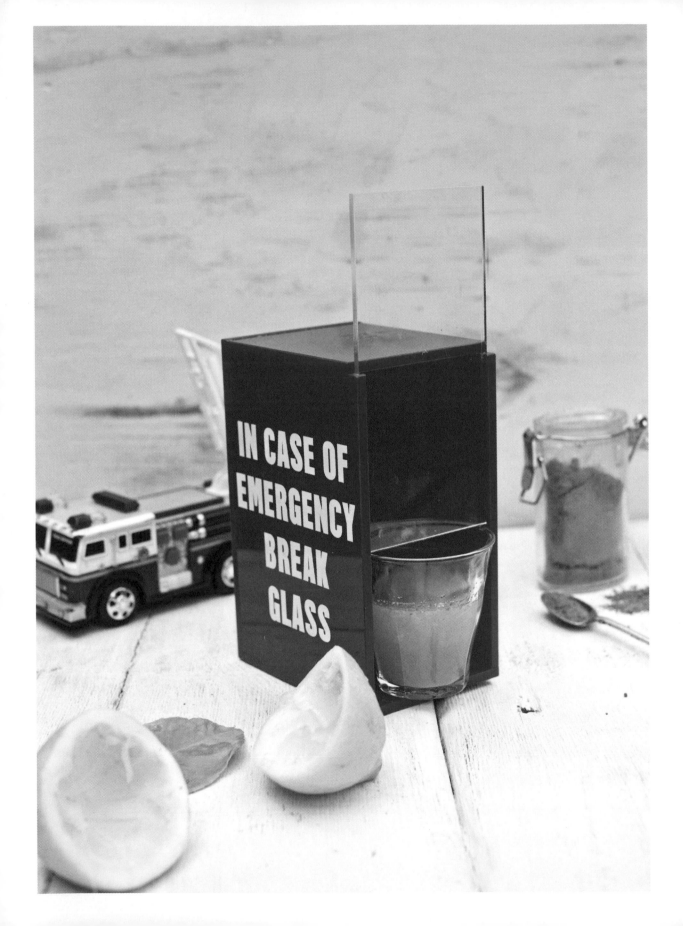

HOT SHOTS

****

Chilli peppers can sting lips to a sumptuous pout without the price tag of cosmetic surgery. Groovy, eh? I guess nettles could too, but I'm not willing to find out. Given that chillies also help raise blood pressure, it's the perfect ingredient to have up your sleeve on a date.

A compound found in this devious little vegetable has been shown to stimulate the release of feel-good endorphins, like a jamboree through the veins. These same endorphins help to put out internal fires by blocking inflammation in the body, numbing us of our day's aches and pains. (And tedious colleagues.)

Historically, chillies were not merely used as an aphrodisiac; they also played a role in alleviating chronic pain and servicing circulatory problems. That's right, gentlemen. Most notably, chilli pepper fortified the chocolate drink that Montezuma the Great consumed to make his pulse dance in preparation for visits to his concubines. No need for little blue pills back then.

This hot shot can help anaesthetise boredom in the boardroom. Although it might also dangerously excite your circulation. Only one way to find out.

Juice the lemons whole or with a citrus presser. Whisk through the raw honey and cayenne. In January and February, Moroccan bergamot lemons are celestial. Find them in grocers and farmers' markets.

Serve in shot glasses or store in the fridge for your hour of need. The lemon shots will stay fresh for two days.

4 lemons
2 tablespoons raw honey
a nip of cayenne pepper

Serves 2-4

LIMONADE

****

Limes are the Sharon Corr of the citrus clan - the elegant, sweet, understated one who has a rhythm all her own. Mojitos made them trendy. Beyoncé made them an industry. And Corona brought them to a different stratosphere. We're loving limes. Lemons were never so yesterday.

This fruit's vitamin C and bioflavonoid content is enough to get beauty queens and cardiologists excited. Both nutrients can help heal zits and plump up tired skin, while a flavonoid called kaempferol has been indicated in the reduction of oxidative damage to our cells. Since oxidised cells can vandalise blood vessels and change cholesterol to make it more likely to build up in artery walls, limes may help to slow down the progression of atherosclerosis. That's doctor speak for sticky arteries.

5 limes
1-2 tablespoons stevia
 Erylite, agave or maple
 syrup
filtered water

Makes 6 servings

Press the limes over a citrus juicer until every last drop is extracted. Add your choice of sweetener and a splash of fresh filtered water. But watch out - honey sinks and stevia is way sweeter than sugar.

Serve in dinky shot glasses. Refrigerate leftovers for up to four days. If you want to serve this with vodka and ice, I'm not going to stop you.

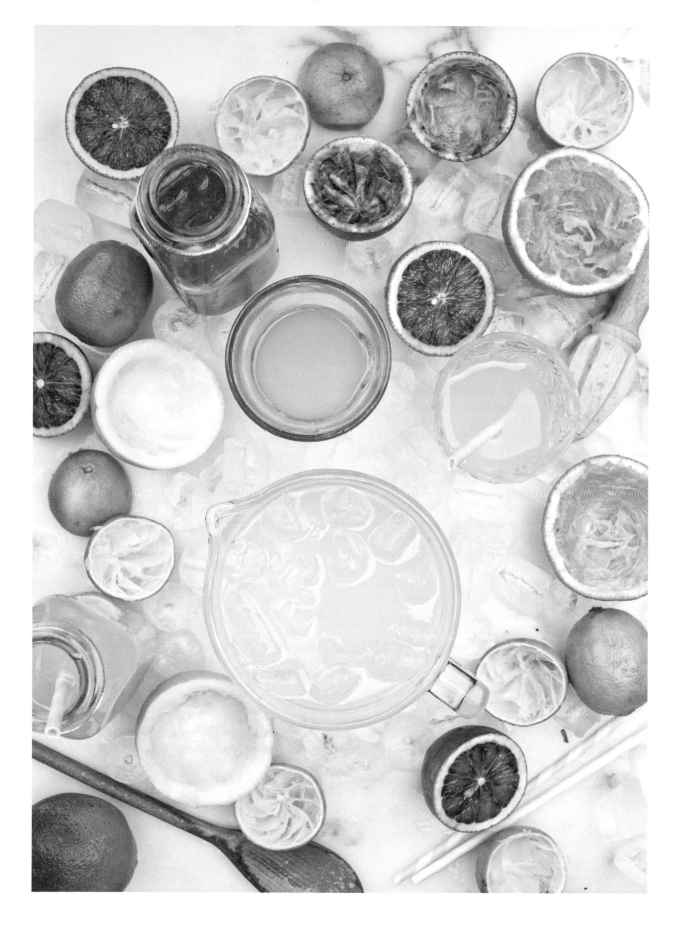

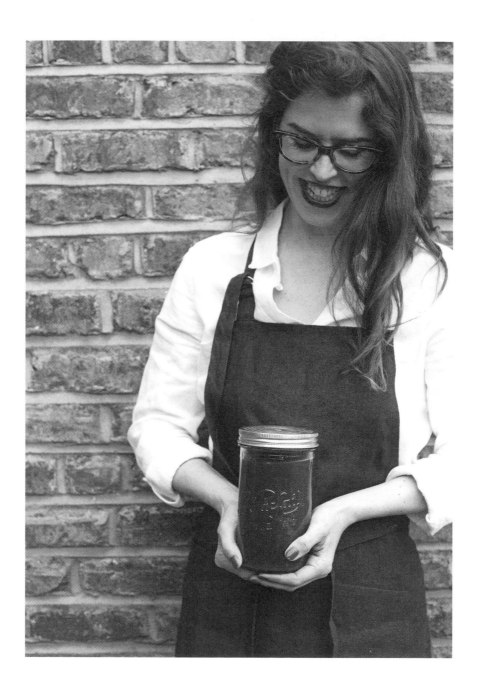

PROBIOTIC COFFEE

****

Coffee addict? This is a game changer, bound to have a seismic effect in your life. The Cultured Club in Belfast taught me how to ferment my own batch of hand-roasted coffee beans, and now the recipe is all yours.

Let the sugar dissolve in the hot coffee. Wait until the sweetened coffee cools before adding your starter culture and the kombucha scoby. I use a 500ml glass Kilner jar for this and secure the top with a piece of muslin instead of a lid.

Leave for 5–10 days. The scoby should have fermented most of the sugar by now and the good bacteria will have multiplied. An ideal environment would be in a dark corner at room temperature. The longer you leave the kombucha to ferment, the tarter it becomes.

As soon as you like the taste, pour 80% of the now-cultured coffee into a clean bottle with a lid and refrigerate for up to two weeks. The remaining 20% is basically your mature kombucha starter for the next batch. You'll notice a baby scoby attached to the mother scoby, which you'll need to discard or compost, otherwise your next batch will be too tart. That's it! Fairly swell, eh?

2 tablespoons coconut or rapadura sugar
2 cups (500ml) hot, fresh filtered coffee
$^{1}/_{4}$ cup (60ml) mature kombucha (see pages 80–81)
1 kombucha scoby (see pages 80–81)

Makes 2 cups (500ml)

2

VIRTUOUS

TURN YOUR CRAVINGS INTO A NUTRITIONAL SLAM-DUNK

TARTS

MILF MUFFINS

xxxxxxxxxxxx

Well I wasn't going to call them millet and teff muffins. Maybe MILF muffins have been invented before, but I ain't brave enough to Google it.

Check out this recipe's armament: chickpeas, teff, raspberries, millet, psyllium, olive oil and almond milk. A balistically good way to foxtrot some goodness into your system. In theory these muffins don't keep longer than two days. In practice, they won't keep longer than two minutes.

up to 1 cup (100-140g)
  coconut sugar or jaggery
$1/2$ cup (75g) teff flour
$1/2$ cup (55g) sorghum (sweet
  millet) flour
$1/2$ cup (55g) chickpea flour
1 $1/2$ teaspoons baking powder
1-2 teaspoons ground ginger
$1/2$ teaspoon salt
palmful of dried mulberries
  (about 30 berries) or 20
  fresh raspberries

**FOR THE PLANT-BASED
'BUTTERMILK':**
1 $1/2$ cups (375ml) almond or
  other plant milk
$1/2$ cup (125ml) extra virgin
  olive oil
2 tablespoons psyllium husks
2 teaspoons vanilla extract

Makes 12 muffins

Preheat the oven to 190°C/170°C fan/375°F. Line a 12-mould muffin or fairy cake tin with cupcake cases.

To make the 'buttermilk', whisk the plant milk, olive oil, psyllium and vanilla with a fork, then leave to rest while you get jiggy with the other ingredients.

In a food processor (or with a whisk and tenacity), blend all the dry ingredients except the berries together so that the baking powder is distributed evenly.

Add the plant 'buttermilk' and beat or purée until smooth. Avoid tasting the batter - wet chickpea flour tastes and smells like cat's pee. The cooked result is awesome though, so do persist! Stir in the berries (mulberries are magnificient).

Divide the dough between the 12 cupcake cases and bake for 28 minutes. When the muffins spring back to the touch, they're ready. Remove from the oven, turn the muffins out of the tray and let them cool on a wire rack.

These are best eaten on the same day, but slather on some chia jam (page 133) to resuscitate them after a few days.

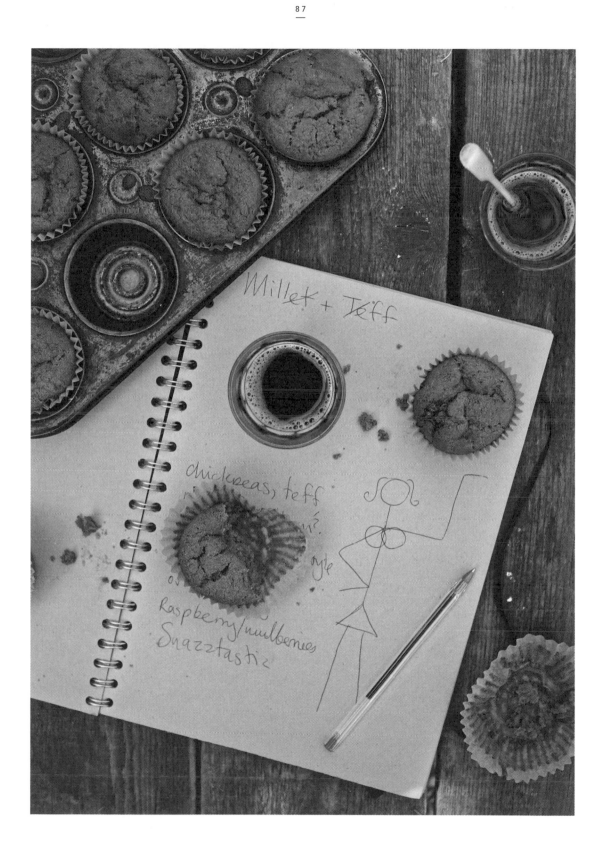

BOOZY CHERRY CUPCAKES

XXXXXXXXXXXXXXXXX

Psyllium husk will make you feel like David Blaine in the kitchen. It transforms grain-free and gluten-free baking. Soak the husks in plant milk to make vegan 'buttermilk'. Barely any chefs and food writers use psyllium, which is a Herculean shame. Let's try to change that.

Similar to slippery elm, psyllium is used to treat both constipation and diarrhoea. How so? The husks of the seed are indigestible and swell to 10 times their weight, creating beneficial mucus for the intestinal tract and lowering transit time (gag). Good for cholesterol too. Rapid. You won't find a better vegan cupcake.

3 tablespoons dried sour cherries
3 tablespoons rum
1 ¹/₂ cups (375ml) almond milk
¹/₂ cup (125ml) extra virgin olive oil
2 tablespoons psyllium husks
1 teaspoon vanilla extract
1 heaped cup (150g) coconut sugar
¹/₂ heaped cup (50g) cocoa or cacao powder
¹/₂ cup (65g) brown rice flour
¹/₂ cup (55g) chestnut flour
¹/₄ cup (40g) potato flour
5 tablespoons (35g) chickpea flour
1 ¹/₂ teaspoons baking powder
¹/₂ teaspoon sea salt flakes

Makes 12 cupcakes

Soak the sour cherries in your rum in a small bowl for between 2 and 48 hours. (You could always use fresh cherries, but I find them dastardly pricey.)

Fire up the oven to 180°C/160°C fan/350°F. Line a 12-mould muffin tin with cupcake cases.

When the cherries are ready to your liking – tart, strong, sweet or offensive – discard the soaking liquid and briskly stir the boozy cherries in with the almond milk, olive oil, psyllium and vanilla. Leave to rest while you introduce yourself to the other ingredients.

In a food processor (or with a whisk and tenacity), blend the coconut sugar, cocoa powder, flours, baking powder and salt together so that the baking powder and cocoa are distributed evenly. Add the boozy wet ingredients and beat until smooth.

Divide the batter between the 12 cupcake liners and bake for 28 minutes. Cool for a few minutes in the tin, then transfer the cupcakes to a wire rack. Inevitably, several will find their way into your mouth. I call this collateral damage. They're especialy good with a sneaky drizzle of melted raw chocolate.

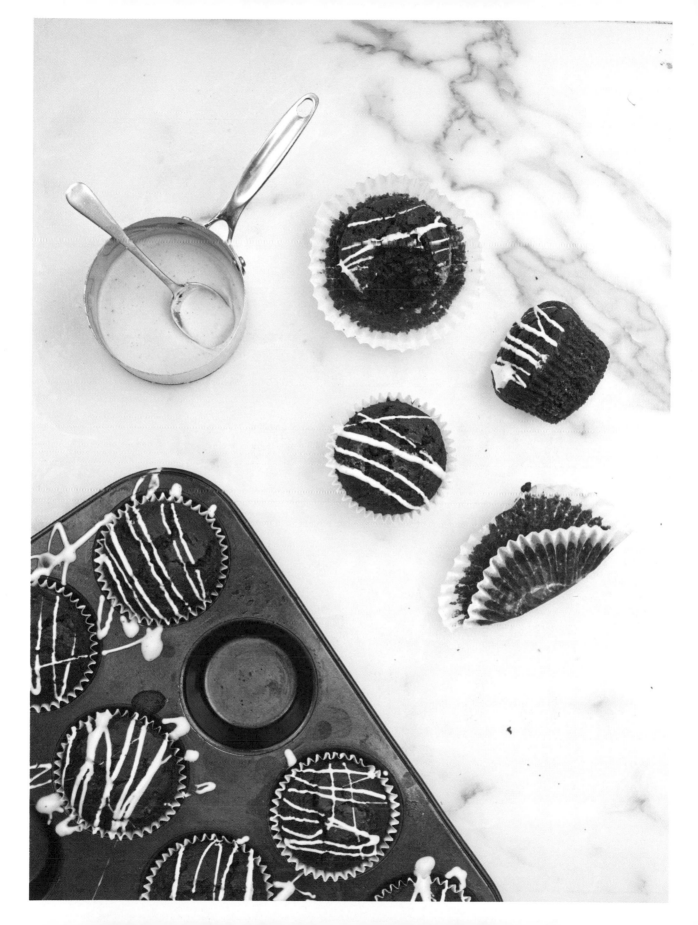

BE
GOOD TO
YOUR BODY.
YOU'RE THE
ONE WHO
HAS TO LIVE
IN IT.

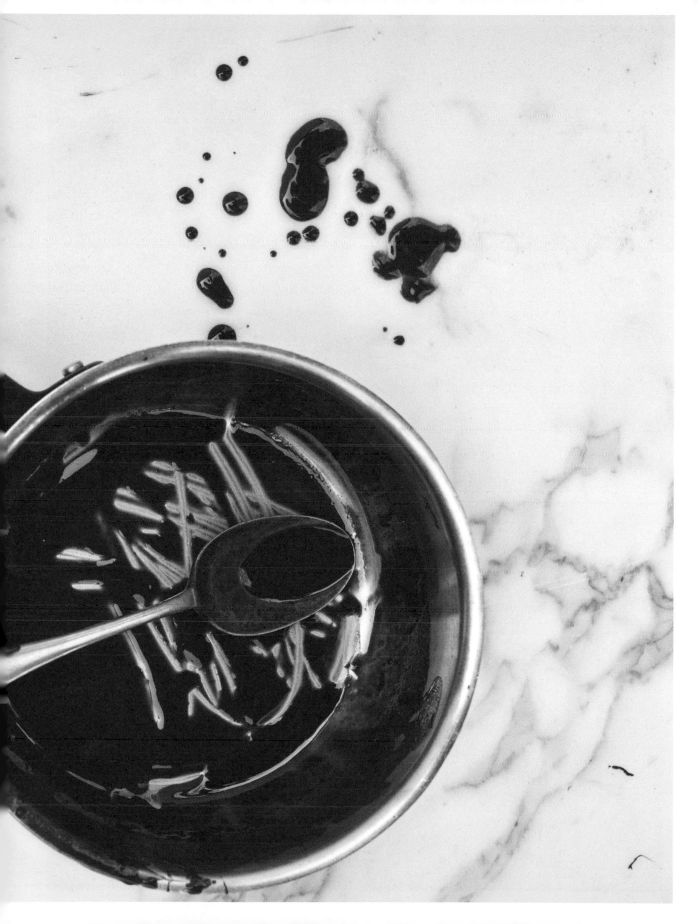

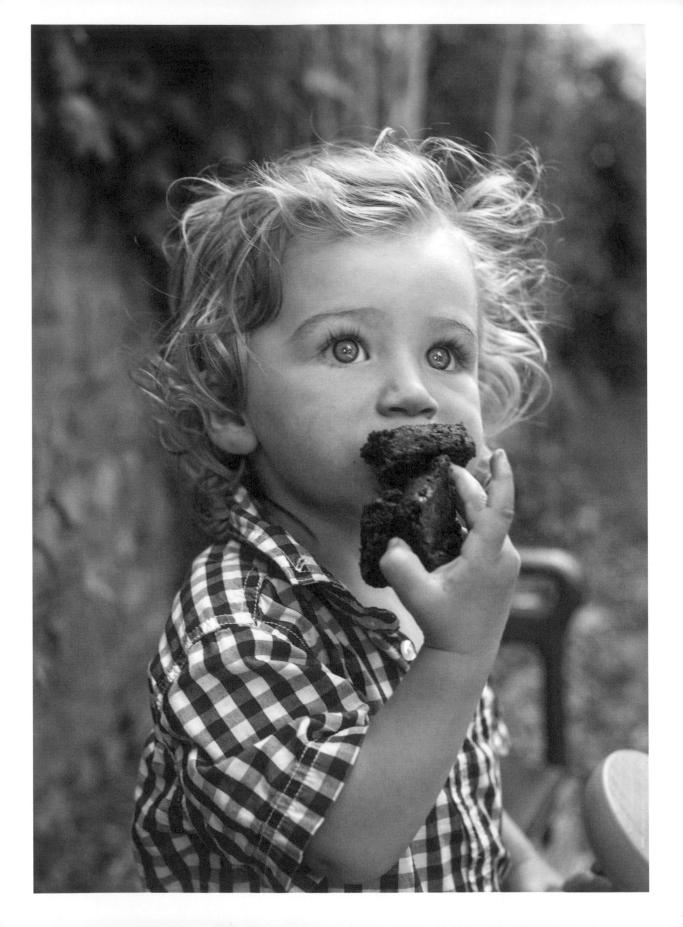

BRAINIAC BROWNIES

xxxxxxxxxxxxxx

When you need to supercharge your poker skills, try chia. These weenchy seeds have finally become mainstream in Ireland, having enjoyed some spectacular adulation across the Atlantic. Everyone from Jessica Alba to David Cameron is tapping into chia mania. Seems like a much more seductive way to get those brain-pumping omega-3s than having to neck fish oil.

First up, make a chia 'egg' by mixing together the almond milk and milled chia seeds in a small bowl. It needs to soak for about 20 minutes.

Preheat the oven to 180°C/160°C fan/350°F. Line a 20cm x 25cm tin with If You Care brand baking parchment to avoid mess and disappointment.

In the meantime, slowly melt the solid block of coconut cream (including the oil on top of the block) with 200g of the dark chocolate in a small saucepan.

In a large bowl, beat the eggs and coconut sugar together until frothy. Stir through the ground almonds and baking powder. Chop up the remaining 25g of chocolate and add it in. Now let the chocolate coconut ganache party with the batter. Finally, drop in your chia 'egg' and a pinch of sea salt flakes. Spoon this glossy gorgeousness into the lined tin.

Bake in the oven for 30 minutes, until you see cracks along the top. Allow to cool in the tin. Best served chilled, when they've had a chance to get fudgy.

$^2/_3$ cup (160ml) almond or other milk
3 tablespoons milled chia seeds
1 block (200g) creamed coconut
225g 70-85% dark chocolate
3 eggs
1 $^1/_2$ cups (210g) coconut sugar
1 cup (100g) ground almonds
2 teaspoons baking powder
good pinch of sea salt flakes

Makes 24 brownies

WTF BROWNIES

xxxxxxxxxx

Raw, pink, vegan brownies with added probiotics. #WTAF.

2 cups (240g) walnuts
1 teaspoon probiotic powder
12 Medjool dates, stones
  removed
6-8 tablespoons cacao or
  cocoa powder
sea salt flakes
2 tablespoons beetroot
  powder, to dust (optional)

Makes 25 brownies

Using a food processor, pulse the walnuts and probiotic powder until they are crumbly.

While the motor is still running, add the Medjool dates down the food processor chute, one by one. It's important to bin the stones first and to check for black dust. If you find that dreaded powdery black stuff, stop the motor. Discard the defected date and any date it happened to socialise with, then wash your hands thoroughly and proceed as usual. Black dust is a sign of plant mould. Guh!

When all the dates have been added, spoon in the cacao or cocoa powder. A generous pinch of sea salt flakes is all that's required now. Give it one last blast in the food processor. Pinch the brownie 'dough' together with your fingertips. If it sticks, you're ready to foxtrot.

Scoop into a lined loaf tin. Press down firmly with the back of a spoon and freeze. After 1-4 hours, remove from the freezer and chop into bite-sized brownies. Return to the freezer in an airtight container. This is where they will live until beckoned. The idea is to eat them straight from frozen. You'll soon understand why. I tell my children they are ice cream brownies and dust them with beetroot powder for their Barbie-loving friends.

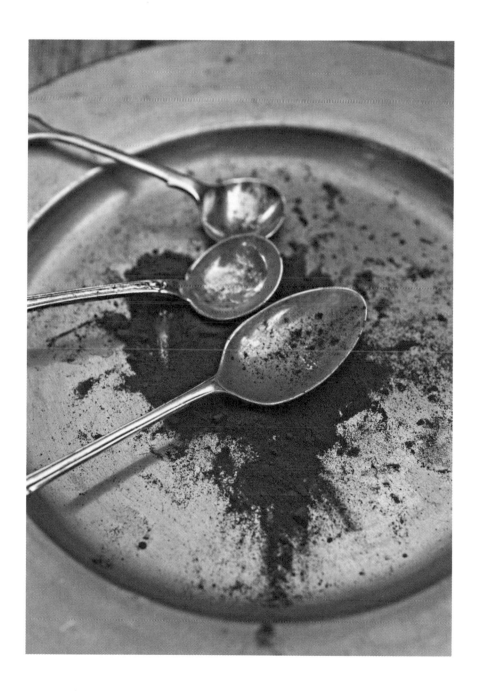

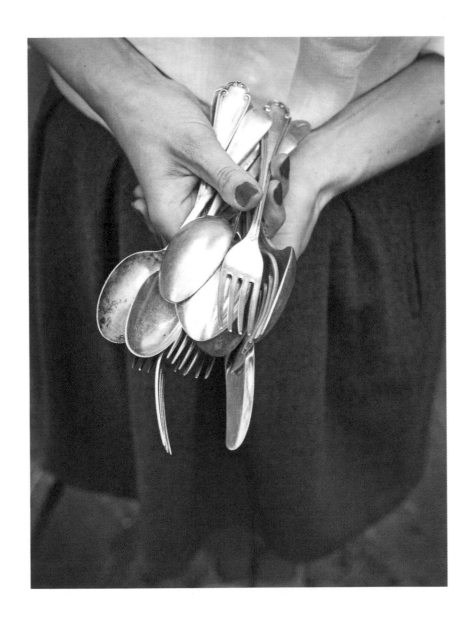

CHOCOLATE GUINNESS CAKE

xxxxxxxxxxxxxxxxxxx

This is St Patrick's Day decadence with a stealthy twist. I cheat by using vacuum-packed beetroot. Don't worry - chocolate sings so loudly, any whisper of vegetable is instantly drowned out. Loaded with beta-carotene, antioxidants and iron, beetroot is famed for its restorative powers on the blood. And anything that helps purify the blood will surely help with hangovers on March 18th. But wait! There's more! Dates are packed with potassium, your ally against hangovers. Potassium is a supersonic mineral that helps rehydrate and jump-start your body again. Not bad for a celebration cake.

Fire up the oven to 180°C/160°C fan/350°F. Grease a 20cm round cake tin or springform tin.

Boil the dates in a small saucepan with the Guinness for 6-8 minutes, until mushy. Purée in a high-speed blender. You're aiming for 1 cup of date paste. Any leftover paste can be stored in the fridge and served with tomorrow's porridge.

Whizz this date paste with the cocoa powder, beetroot purée, coconut flour and tamari until glossy and gorgeous. Blend in the eggs, oil or butter, baking powder and vanilla extract until sumptuous. Immediately pour the batter into your greased tin.

Once the cake is in the oven, lower the heat to 170°C/150°C fan/340°F. This is an important step. I strongly recommend using an oven thermometer when baking, to be sure to be sure. Bake for 45-55 minutes, depending how wet the beetroot was. You're looking for a moist, rich cake, not a dry, fluffy one.

Remove from the oven and allow to cool. Make sure you give the cake enough time to cool down before carefully removing it from the tin. Springform tins are great because the sides just pop off when you release the clip.

Using a big spoon, slather the yoghurt over the top of the chocolate cake to resemble a pint of Guinness.

Happy Paddy's Day!

2 heaped cups (300g) regular pitted dates
1 cup (250ml) Guinness stout
1 1/4 cups (125g) cocoa powder
1 cup (250ml) puréed beetroot (about 4 cooked baby beets from a vacuum packet)
1/4 cup (30g) coconut flour
2 teaspoons tamari soya sauce
4 medium eggs
1/2 cup (125ml) extra virgin olive oil or melted butter
2 teaspoons baking powder
2 teaspoons vanilla extract
up to 1 cup (350g) Greek or coconut milk yoghurt (page 130)

Makes 24 servings

BANOFFEE MESS

xxxxxxxxxxxx

Sleep deprivation is the latest tax to hit us. Quite apart from nights lost to insatiable Visa bills and episodes of The Killing, everyone seems to be popping babies. Look out for dazed brethren roaming our office corridors and streets. Should you spot one, approach with caution and slip them a copy of this recipe.

The key to optimising your chances of a smooth trip to Slumberville is replenishing your reserves of zinc and vitamin B6 in your diet. Both are crucial for the production of your brain's sleepy hormone, melatonin. No B6 or zinc, no zeds.

Stress drinks up our banks of zinc and B6, resulting in a deficiency at night. No one functions well on a poor night's sleep. Not even Mary Poppins. Our concentration falls, our patience wheezes and our immunity chokes. Of course, ditching caffeine and taking up meditation is the most effective way of repairing adrenal glands. But for most of us, such a proposal is enough to detonate our stress levels.

So who would have thought that a twist on the classic banoffee pie could help? Bananas contain vitamin B6 and the mineral zinc can be sourced from the pecans in this recipe. I recommend investing in some quality time with these foods before booking into a fancy hypnosis centre or resorting to Celine Dion's greatest hits.

1 ¹/₂ cups (210g) regular pitted dates
¹/₂ cup (140g) cashew nut butter
3 tablespoons lúcuma powder or 1 teaspoon vanilla extract
1 tablespoon unscented coconut oil
good pinch of sea salt flakes
1 cup (250g) regular or coconut milk yoghurt (page 130)
3 bananas, sliced
4 squares of dark chocolate
toasted pecans (page 174)

Serves 6

Cover the dates with a little water in a small saucepan and boil for 10 minutes. Whip in a food processor with the cashew nut butter, lúcuma or vanilla, coconut oil and a good pinch of sea salt until seriously smooth. Allow to cool down before you judge! At this stage, it won't taste or smell like caramel.

Scoop some yoghurt into six little pots. Add a few slices of fresh banana, followed by a glossy kiss of the caramel. Top with optional shavings of dark chocolate if you have some. No biggie if not. Toasted pecans scattered on top give a great crunch.

Serve to unsuspecting guests and see if they notice the difference.

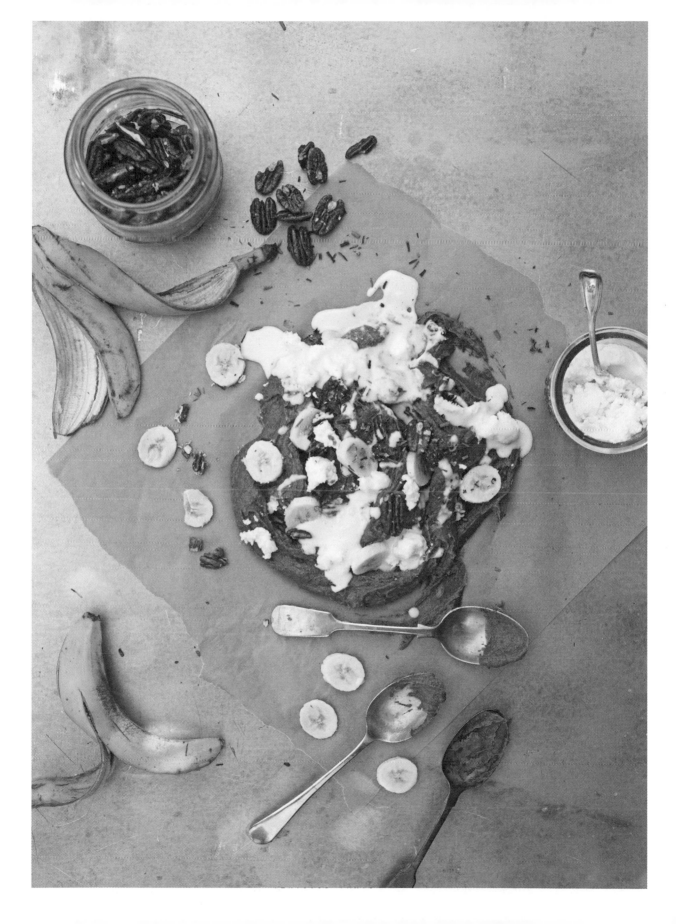

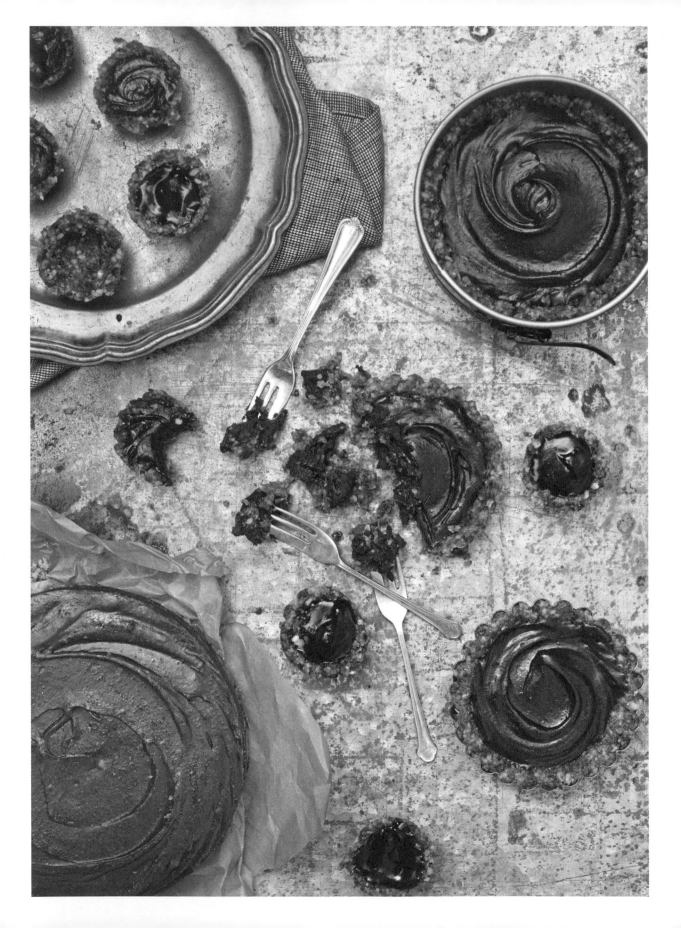

EARL GREY CHOCOLATE TARTLETS

×××××××××××××××××××××××

Can we fight cancer with a fork? Dr William Li thinks we can. His research team has discovered a range of foods that inhibit the blood supply to cancer, effectively slowing or stopping the cancer's growth. Li's work demonstrates that the bigger the supply of blood vessels to the tumour, the quicker the cancer will grow. He refers to this as angiogenesis.

Li suggests we increase certain foods in our diet to naturally inhibit the blood supply to cancerous cells. He calls these antiangiogenesis foods. Li's list includes red grapes, green tea, Earl Grey tea, strawberries, parsley, artichokes, garlic and cooked tomatoes (all terribly tasty). And guess what? Every ingredient in this tart is listed as antiangiogenic.

Dear Pope Francis, I concede. There is a God.

To make the base, pulse the walnuts with the chopped dates and salt. You might need the teeniest splash of water to bring it together.

Press the mixture firmly into a dinky tray of small cupcake holders. Silicone ones are best because the mixture won't stick. Cookie cutters are useful too. Line the sides and the bottom as thinly as you can. Freeze. You can also use three 8cm pans or one 18cm springform cake pan instead if it all seems too tedious.

To make the filling, give the cashew butter, avocado (if using), hot water, cacao powder, maple syrup and tamari a good whizz in the blender. You should have a dense, dark, glossy ganache by now. While the motor is running, slowly add a steady stream of melted cacao butter and four drops of bergamot oil. Taste and decide whether you'd like more sweetness or perhaps more saltiness from the tamari.

Once you're happy, spoon the filling into each of your prepped cupcake holders and smooth the top with your tongue or spoon, whichever is more appealing. If you have any filling left over, scrape it into silicone ice cube trays and freeze for 10 minutes. Instant raw chocolates!

I store my platoon of tartlets in the freezer, ready to serve at late notice with little strips of orange peel if I have it. The mini ones are useful for parties and pass-arounds.

FOR THE BASE:
1 2/3 cups (180g) walnuts
3/4 cup (110g) Medjool dates, pitted and chopped
pinch of sea salt flakes

FOR THE FILLING:
1 1/2 cups (1/0g) cashew or hazelnut butter
1/2 very ripe avocado (optional)
1/4 cup (60ml) hot water
6 tablespoons raw cacao or cocoa powder
5 tablespoons maple syrup
2-3 teaspoons tamari soya sauce
3 tablespoons melted cacao butter
4 drops of culinary-grade bergamot oil (this is what makes Earl Grey tea)

Makes 12-18 tartlets for the freezer

MACACCINO TORTE WITH TOASTED PECAN AND CHOCOLATE CRUMB

xxxxxxxxxxxxxxxxxxxxxxxxxxxxxxxxxxxxxxxxxxxxxxxxx

Maca is the Lucozade of the granola-crunching, wheatgrass-swilling community. This golden fairy dust is supposed to strengthen stamina and virility, so keep it away from the teens.

I've noticed that people who scoff maca are already health-conscious, athletic specimens with a sex drive that makes Silvio Berlusconi look impotent. I can't accuse maca of causing the latest baby boom, but I'm always partial to a rigorous experiment.

Did you know that the more saucy sessions we indulge in, the more stress-relieving endorphins we release? These endorphins help strengthen our immune system too. So nookie is our inbuilt superfood. Win-win!

If you're curious, this mystical maca comes in powdered form resembling a sort of butterscotch flour. It's fun to use, and if it does indeed boost libido, then it's even more fun than I expected. Good luck.

FOR THE BASE:
1 cup (110g) pecans
5 Medjool dates or pre-
   soaked regular dates,
   pitted and chopped
2 tablespoons cacao or cocoa
   powder
sprinkle of sea salt flakes

FOR THE CREAM FILLING:
1 1/2 cups (170g) cashew nut
   butter
6 tablespoons maple syrup or
   coconut blossom nectar
5 tablespoons hot, strong
   coffee
3 tablespoons maca powder
2 tablespoons lúcuma powder
   or 1 teaspoon vanilla
   extract
2-3 teaspoons tamari soya
   sauce
4 tablespoons melted cacao
   butter
4-5 squares of dark
   chocolate, melted, to
   decorate
coffee beans, to decorate
   (optional)

Makes 20 servings

To make the base, put all the base ingredients in a food processor and whizz together until they begin to clump into a ball. You might need the tiniest trickle of cold water or coffee to bring it together, depending on how soft the dates are. I like to toast my pecans first (see page 174), but it's not necessary.

Press the mixture firmly into a non-stick 18cm springform tin or whatever torte flan you have. Set in the freezer while you get going on the cream filling.

To make the filling, give the cashew butter, maple syrup, hot coffee, maca, lúcuma and tamari a good pelt in a high-speed blender or food processor. Don't feel you need to buy lúcuma especially for this recipe. A dash of vanilla will work just as well, but I happen to worship the buttery, caramel tones of lúcuma.

Slowly add the melted cacao butter to the mix while the motor is still running. You should have a glossy maca-fuelled ganache by now. Spread the filling over your base and refrigerate until set. You can happily keep this macaccino torte in the freezer too, for unexpected dates.

To decorate, go mad with melted dark chocolate and a spoon and parachute some coffee beans on top.

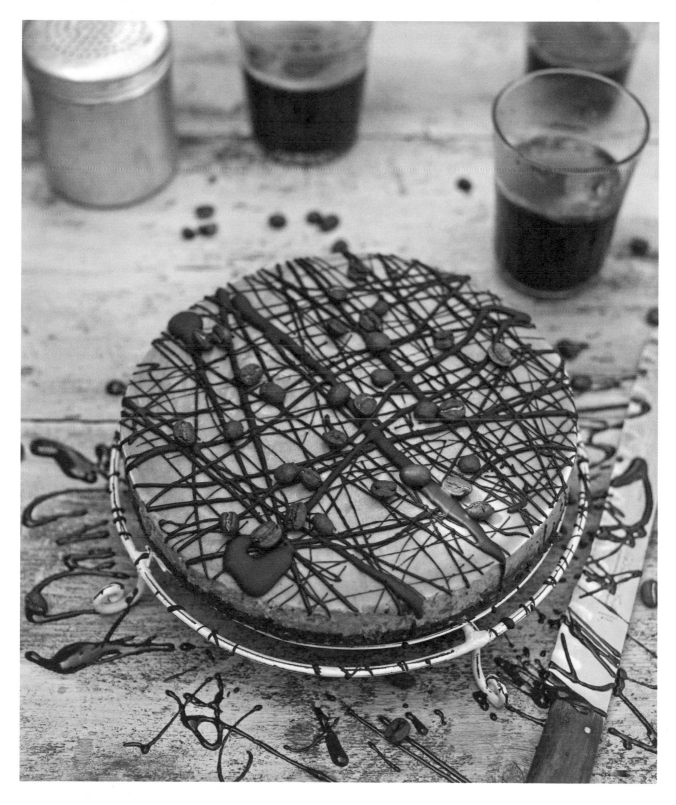

VIRTUOUS TARTS

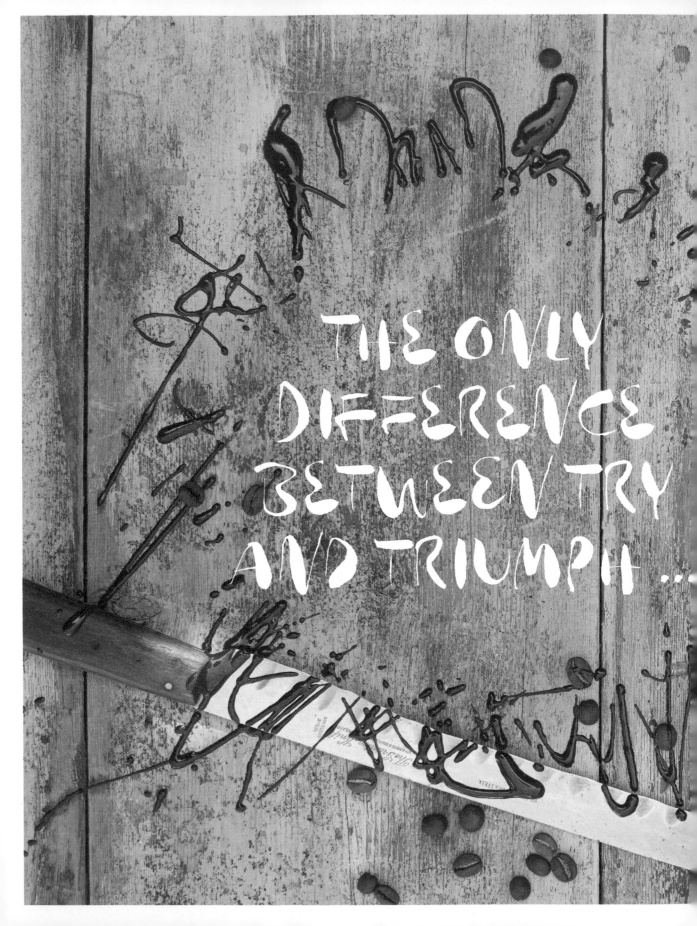

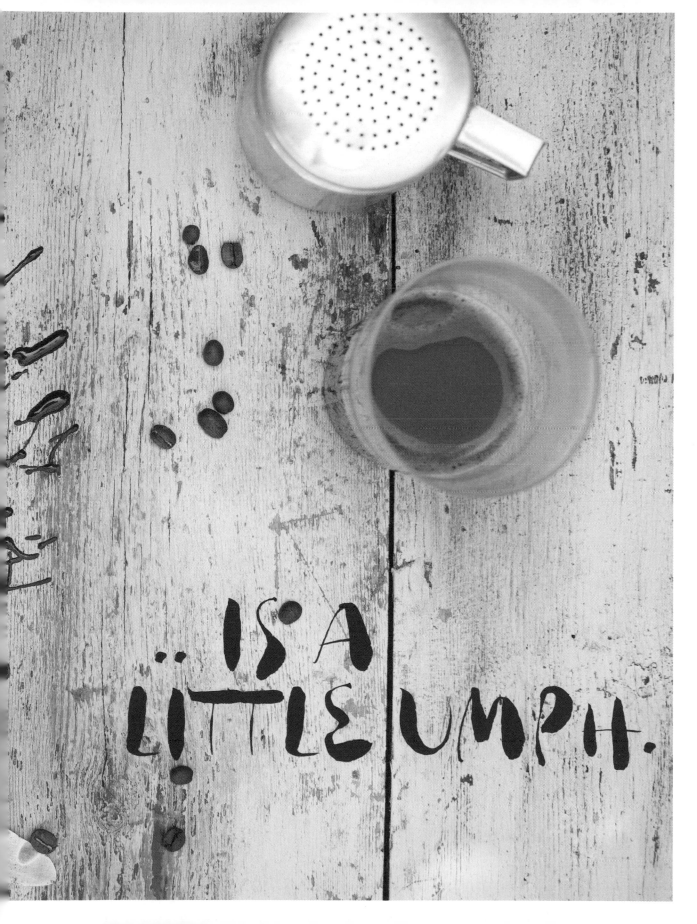

... IS A
LITTLE UMPH.

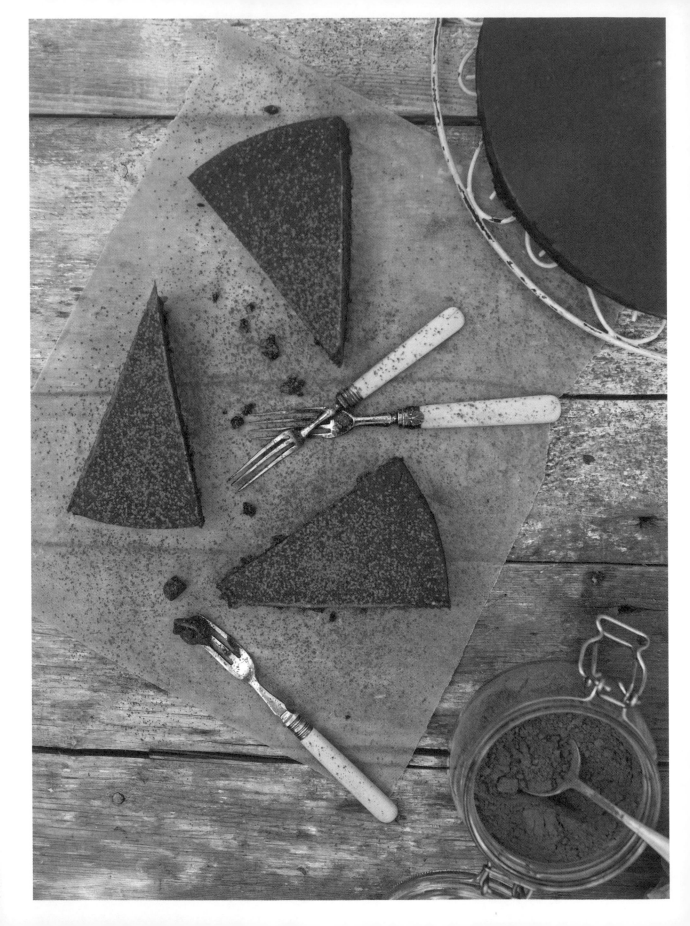

AFTER EIGHT DINNER PARTY TORTE

xxxxxxxxxxxxxxxxxxxxxxxxxx

The mere whiff of cacao butter sends a cavalry of hormones pelting through my veins like a pinball machine. My chest swells and my nostrils levitate. It would be a tragedy to miss out on a cacao butter head rush. You think I'm joking? I get regular bulk deliveries and squeal louder than a One Direction front-row fan when the courier calls. This is a fierce twist on a classic.

To make the base, tumble the nuts, dates, cacao powder and a pinch of salt into a food processor and pulse until crumbly but sticky. You will need the teeniest splash of water to bring it together. Press the mixture firmly into an 18cm springform tin (you'll find these on Amazon). Refrigerate.

To make the filling, give the cashew butter, hot water, maple syrup, cacao powder, tamari and peppermint a good whizz in the food processor. Every brand of peppermint oil has a different intensity, so start small (three drops) and work up to six if necessary. Slowly add the melted cacao butter. You should have a dense, dark, glossy ganache by now. Taste and decide whether you'd like more peppermint, but too much will taste like mouth wash.

Once you're happy, spread the filling over your base and decorate with fresh mint leaves. Store in the freezer, or your belly.

FOR THE BASE:
1 1/2 cups (180g) walnuts
  and/or pecans
1/2 cup (75g) Medjool dates,
  pitted and chopped
1 tablespoon raw cacao or
  cocoa powder
pinch of organic unrefined
  salt

FOR THE FILLING:
2/3 cup (190g) cashew nut
  butter
6 tablespoons hot water
6 tablespoons maple syrup or
  coconut nectar (maple is
  sweeter)
5 tablespoons raw cacao or
  cocoa powder
2 teaspoons tamari soya
  sauce
3-6 drops of culinary
  grade peppermint oil or
  1/2 teaspoon peppermint
  extract
4 tablespoons melted cacao
  butter
fresh mint leaves, to
  decorate

Makes 24 servings

PRESSED COCONUT TORTE WITH TAMARIND AND MISO CARAMEL

xxxxxxxxxxxxxxxxxxxxxxxxxxxxxxxxxxxxxxxxxxxxxxxx

I reckon this torte is the tastiest thing to hit our cosmology in a long time (excluding you, Bradley Cooper). No baking involved. Just a lot of adulation.

Tamarind is Mother Nature's sherbet - sour, sweet and tart. Just like unicorn tears (don't ask). If you can't get sweet white miso, use any miso paste you fancy but use half the amount. Or replace with scrumptious sea salt flakes.

FOR THE BASE:
1 cup (120g) walnuts
6 Medjool dates, stones
  removed
1 tablespoon cocoa powder
pinch of sea salt flakes

FOR THE FILLING:
3 cups (240g) desiccated
  coconut
6-8 tablespoons brown rice
  syrup or light agave
5 tablespoons (75ml) extra
  virgin coconut oil

FOR THE CARAMEL:
1 cup (150g) regular pitted
  dates
$1/3$ cup (95g) cashew butter
4 teaspoons sweet white miso
4 teaspoons sticky fresh
  tamarind

FOR THE CRUNCH:
5 squares of dark chocolate,
  melted

Makes 16-18 servings

To make the base, oil an 18cm springform tin. Pulse all the base ingredients in a food processor rather than a blender. The food processor blade will chop it all up and press the mixture together without turning it into a paste. Scrape into the oiled tin. You can flatten it fairly swiftly if you use a sheet of baking parchment between your fingers and the mixture - it's very sticky. Freeze the base while you get to work on the filling.

To make the filling, blend the desiccated coconut with your choice of syrup and the coconut oil in a high-speed processor for 4-5 minutes. You're looking for a buttery, spreadable consistency. Maple syrup and coconut blossom nectar will turn the torte brown, so bear this in mind if you're trying to substitute them for the brown rice syrup or agave. It will still taste amazeballs. Spread over the frozen base and return to the freezer until set (approximately 1 hour).

To make the tamarind and miso caramel, cover the dates with a little water and boil in a small saucepan for 10 minutes. Whip in a food processor with the cashew nut butter, miso and tamarind until smooth and shiny. Allow to cool down before you judge the flavour, because at this stage it won't taste or smell like caramel. I usually add a little warm water to thin it out.

Spread the caramel on top of the coconut filling, followed by flecks of melted chocolate. Or serve the caramel in place of cream in a little jug. Let your eyes decide.

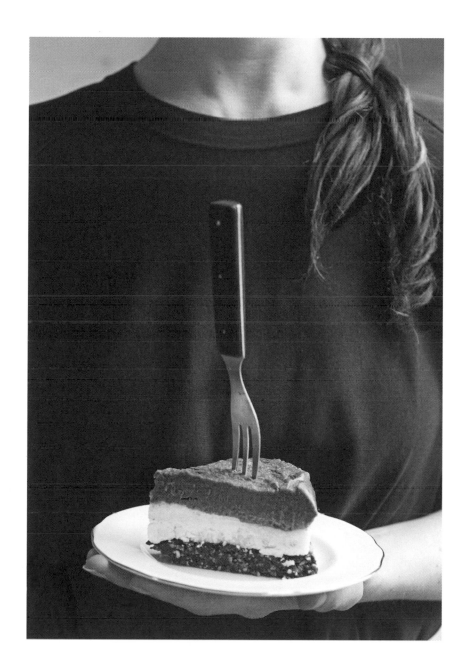

VIRTUOUS TARTS

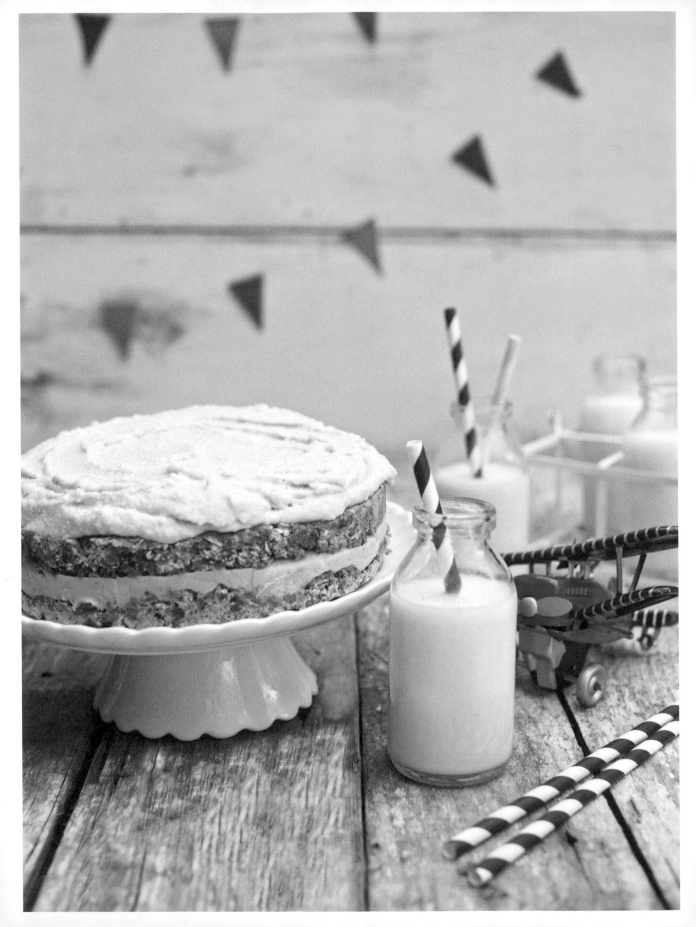

RAWVOLUTIONARY CARROT CAKE

xxxxxxxxxxxxxxxxxxxxxx

I freeze the entire cake in nifty slices, ready for their call of duty. One slice will fill your sails. Expect an afternoon glow to rival that of Saoirse Ronan at the Oscars.

Insoluble fibre has the crafty ability to police our bowels, improving congestion and reducing transit time like a tenacious traffic warden. Oats and dried fruit contain astral amounts of the stuff. Oats have additional bragging rights - all those B vitamins will help recharge spent batteries and frayed nerves, while slow-release carbs will have your toes cha-cha-ing all day long. For more rawesome inspiration, check out Emily von Euw faster than immediately.

The frosting comes first. Soak the cashews and pine nuts in a large bowl of filtered water for 6 hours or overnight.

In the morning, drain and rinse the soaked nuts. Tumble into a blender with the remaining frosting ingredients (except the pumpkin seeds) and purée until smooth. You may need an extra bit of juice to loosen it up to a spreadable consistency. Leave aside for now.

Then make the cake. Grate the carrots into your food processer (blenders are too powerful), then tip in the remaining cake ingredients. Pulse until it starts sticking. Taste and high five Mother Nature.

Scrape half of the cake mixture into an 18cm springform tin and press down firmly. Spread half of the frosting on top. Freeze for 30 minutes, until firm. Now spoon in the remaining carrot mixture on top of the frozen cake, press down and top with the remaining frosting. Freeze again.

Store in the freezer in its tin until ready to serve. At this point, carefully remove the cake from the springform tin by manipulating the sides and the base. I sometimes double up on frosting and cover the entire beast, parachuting some pumpkin seeds on top. Fandabbydoozy.

FOR THE FROSTING:
1 cup (135g) cashews
1/2 cup (70g) pine nuts (or more cashews)
1/2 cup (125ml) light agave nectar or raw honey
3 tablespoons freshly squeezed orange juice
2 tablespoons freshly squeezed lemon juice
1 tablespoon finely minced fresh ginger
scrape of orange zest
pumpkin seeds, to decorate

FOR THE CAKE:
275g carrots, peeled and grated (2 big carrots)
1 1/2 cups (135g) oat flakes
1 cup (140g) regular pitted dates, chopped
1 cup (50g) unsweetened dried pineapple
1/2 cup (40g) desiccated coconut
palmful of raisins
2 tablespoons maca
1 tablespoon water
1 teaspoon ground cinnamon
1 teaspoon ground turmeric
pinch of sea salt flakes
squeeze of lemon juice

Makes 20 servings

VICTORIA SPONGE WITH CHIA JAM AND COCONUT CREAM

XXXXXXXXXXXXXXXXXXXXXXXXXXXXXXXXXXXXXXXX

Not the traditional butter, cream, sugar and bleached-flour variety, this Victoria sponge will make your taste buds backflip and your health insurer applaud. Make it for a group of Brits and you'll have friends for life.

FOR THE SPONGE:

¹/₂ cup (65g) coconut flour
1 teaspoon baking powder
¹/₄ cup (25g) ground almonds
¹/₄ teaspoon mineral-rich salt, like pink Himalayan
4 medium (not large) eggs
2 tablespoons natural or soya yoghurt
1 teaspoon vanilla extract
¹/₂ cup (125ml) light agave, brown rice syrup or honey (honey is much sweeter than brown rice syrup)
just under ¹/₂ cup (120ml) unscented coconut oil, melted, plus extra for greasing
1 tablespoon freshly squeezed lemon juice

FOR THE FILLING:

²/₃ cup (125g) frozen raspberries, defrosted
3 Medjool dates, stones removed
1-2 tablespoons chia seeds
squeeze of lime juice
4–8 tablespoons coconut milk yoghurt (page 130)

Makes 10 portions (double to serve 20)

To make the chia jam filling, whizz the thawed raspberries in a food processor or hand-held blender with the licky-sticky dates, chia seeds and lime juice. Allow the chia seeds to thicken the jam for 40 minutes before using.

Preheat your oven to 170°C/150°C fan/340°F. You'll need to oil a 20cm x 20cm square brownie tin. I find the best oil to use for greasing is unscented (as opposed to extra virgin and raw) coconut oil. Unscented coconut oil won't turn the edges of the sponge infuriatingly dark. The meat of the coconut is lightly steamed before being pressed in order to remove the strong coconutty aroma from the oil.

To make the cake, take out two large bowls. In the first bowl, sift your coconut flour with the baking powder. Stir through the ground almonds and the salt.

In the next bowl, whisk the eggs and yoghurt together, adding a splash of vanilla extract. Then pour in the sweetener and melted coconut oil, stirring vigorously to prevent lumps. Gradually drizzle in the lemon juice, whisking all the while. Scrape this gleefully sticky mess into your prepared tin and level with a spatula.

Bake for 20 minutes. Remove the sponge from the oven before the edges darken. Let it cool on a wire rack for 1 hour before ejecting from the tin. Then carefully slice the sponge in half to make two layers (of course, you could always double the recipe and make two big tiers instead). Smother great big clouds of coconut milk yoghurt over one half. Parachute a little chia jam on top of this, then crown with the other half of the sponge. Serve on a plate with many napkins and giddy fingers. And a side of Sinatra.

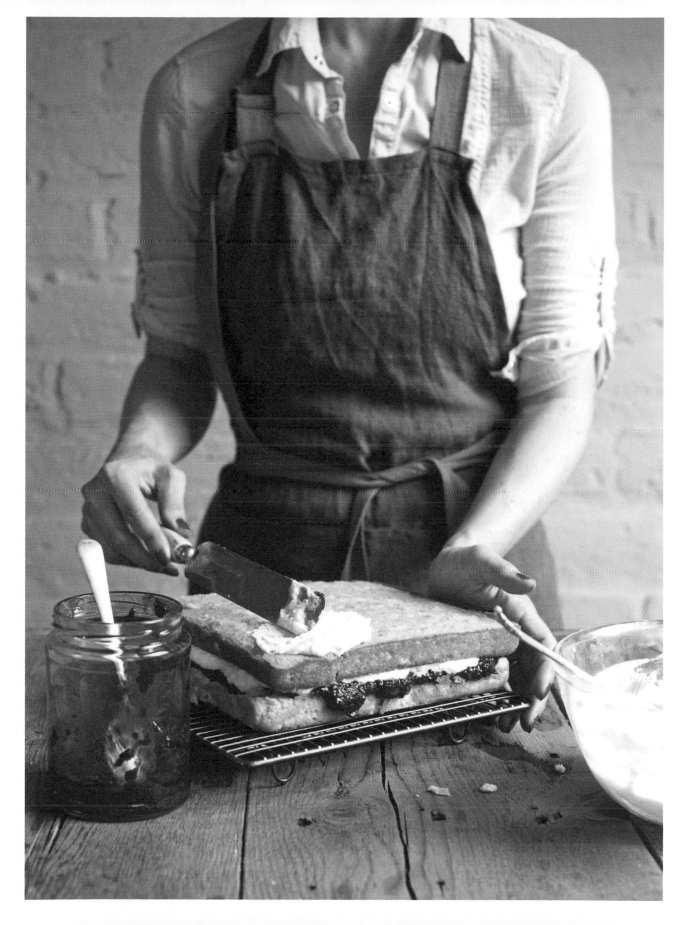

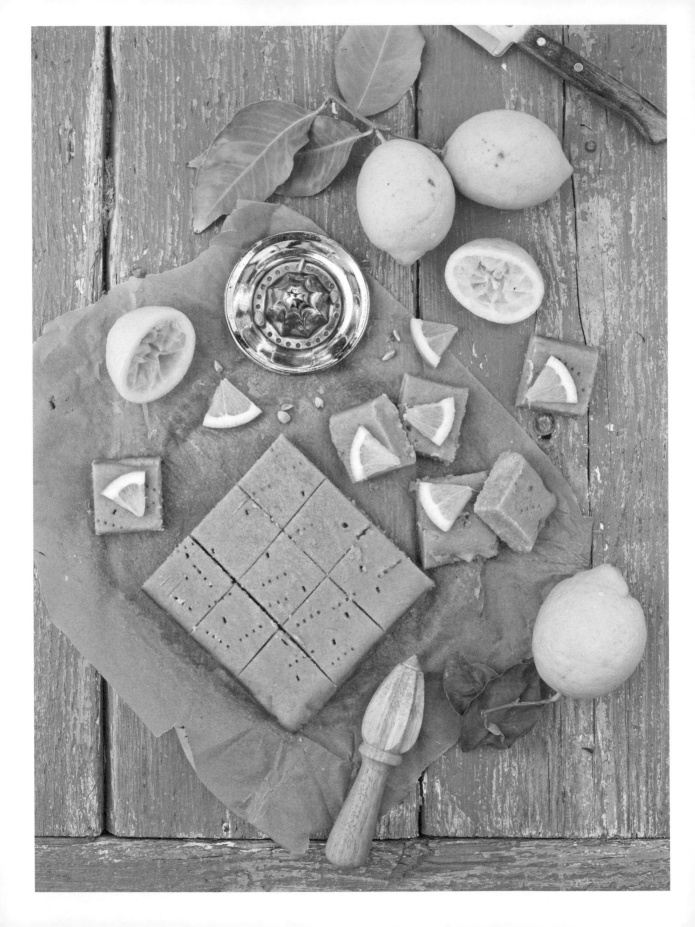

LEMON SHIZZLE CAKE

xxxxxxxxxxxxxxx

This sticky citrus cake is practically belching with age-defying vitamins like E, C and plant-based calcium. Its fantastical glow comes from a spice called turmeric, also known as poor man's saffron. Turmeric delivers a cargo of anti-inflammatory artillery for squeaky bones and damaged skin. Think of it as Botox baking.

Preheat the oven to 170°C/150°C fan/340°F. Line a 20cm x 20cm square brownie tin with non-stick paper, such as the If You Care brand (the best on the market – see page 201).

Blend everything in a food processor or electric blender. That's it!

Pour into your prepped tin and bake for 22-25 minutes, removing it from the oven before it browns. Leave to cool in the tin.

Now for the shizzle. Gently warm the lemon juice with the agave or honey in a small saucepan. Taste test. Add more sweetener if it seems alarmingly tart. Pour over your cake while still warm. A few piercings from a fork will help. Admire your brilliance and let your nostrils samba.

3 cups (300g) ground almonds
4 eggs
juice of 1 large unwaxed
  lemon
6 tablespoons cold-pressed
  macadamia or coconut oil
up to 3 tablespoons light
  agave or honey
1 teaspoon baking powder
1 teaspoon ground turmeric
¹/₂ teaspoon unrefined salt

FOR THE DRIZZLE:
juice of 1 lemon
approx. 2 tablespoons light
  agave or raw honey

Makes 16 servings

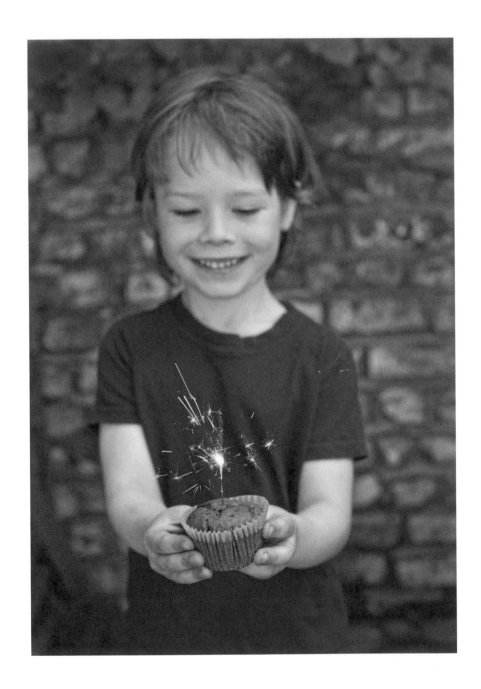

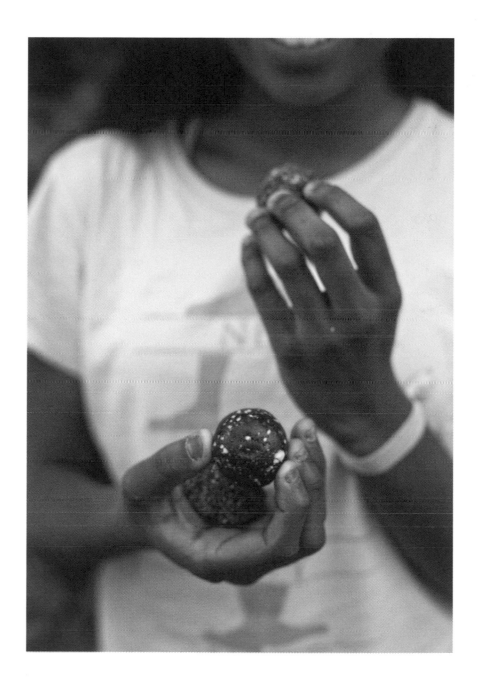

VIRTUOUS TARTS

ORANGE, CARDAMOM AND POLENTA CAKE

xxxxxxxxxxxxxxxxxxxxxxxxxxxx

This is one very special cake, lightly adapted from my favourite chef's kitchen. Forgive me, Nige.

Xylitol sounds like a nuclear bunion buster. It is, in fact, a sweetener derived from the birch tree and is often referred to as birch sugar (see its profile on page 17).

Don't ignore the cardamom seeds - it would be like making brownies without chocolate.

FOR THE CAKE:
1 cup (220g) coconut oil
  (firm, not melted)
1 cup (200g) xylitol birch
  sugar
3 cups (300g) ground almonds
just under 1 cup (150g)
  instant polenta
3 eggs
juice and zest of 2 medium
  unwaxed oranges
12 green cardamom pods,
  seeds only
4 apricot kernels, very
  finely chopped or milled
  (only if you have them)
1 teaspoon baking powder
decent pinch of sea salt
  flakes

FOR THE SYRUP:
juice of 2 small lemons
juice of 2 medium oranges
3–4 tablespoons honey, agave
  or maple syrup

Greek yoghurt or coconut
  milk yoghurt (page 130),
  to serve

Makes 12-16 servings

Fire up your oven to 180°C/160°C fan/350°F. You'll need to grease a 20cm round springform tin for this cake. It's fairly massive.

Using a blender or food processor, cream the coconut oil and xylitol together. Add the remaining cake ingredients and blend until smooth. Spoon into your prepared tin and smooth the top with a spoon or tongue.

Bake for 20 minutes, then reduce the oven temperature to 160°C/140°C fan/325°F for another 40 minutes. You'll know it's done when a skewer comes out clean from the centre of the cake. If the skewer is gooey, it needs longer. But if the skewer only has a few rich crumbs stuck to it after inserting it through the centre, you're done.

As soon as she's out of the oven, make the sticky syrup. Boil the lemon and orange juice with your preferred sweetener until the syrup is somewhat thicker than water - 10 minutes should do the trick. Prod little holes all over the cake, still in its tin, with a metal skewer. Spoon over the hot citrus syrup and watch the cake drink up every drop. Allow to cool for a further 60 minutes before slicing into thick wedges and serving with Greek yoghurt or thick coconut milk yoghurt. Unimaginably delicious.

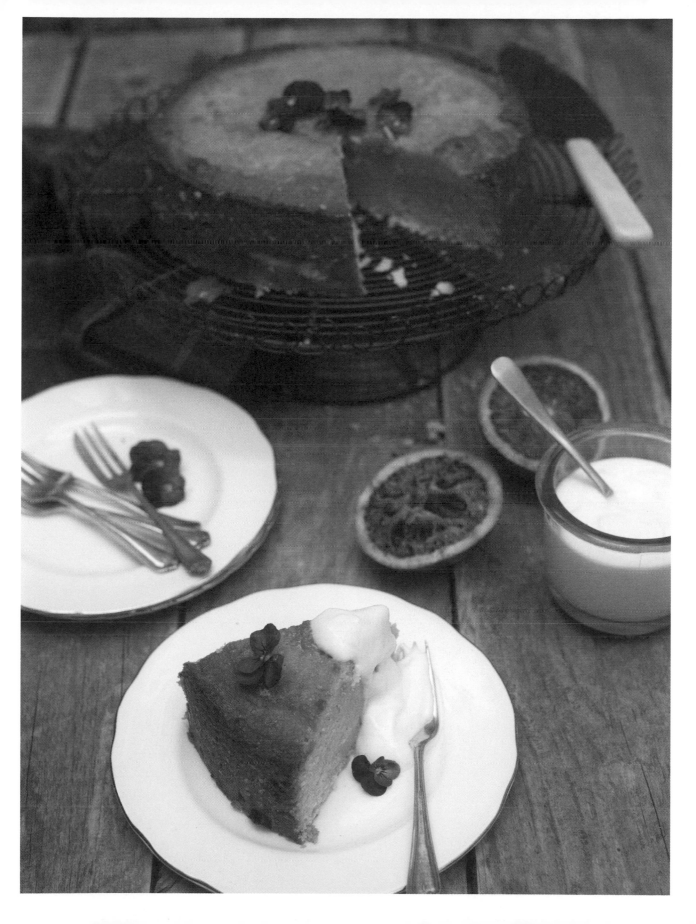

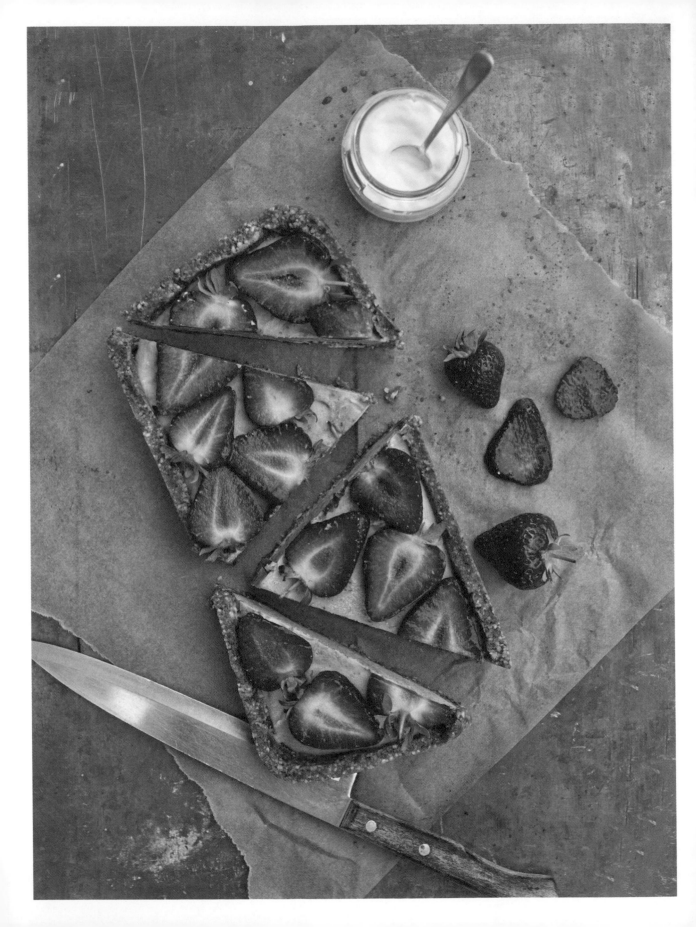

STRAWBERRY AND BASIL CHEESECAKE

XXXXXXXXXXXXXXXXXXXXXXXXX

By loading more fresh veg and nuts into us ladies, we'll arm our bodies against The Ageing Process and give Laura Whitmore some competition. This cake should help. Avocados and almonds are drenched with helpful fats and nourishing minerals needed to keep our toes tapping and skin glowing.

Remember, the skin is your largest excretory organ. If you're eating garbage, you'll end up wearing it in your face.

To make the base, blend the walnuts, dates and sea salt in a food processor (not a blender) with a splash of water. When it starts clumping together into a cookie dough ball, you're good to go. Press into a 20–25cm loaf tin. Bring the dough up the sides like a posh flan, making sure you support the elbow of the base – the part where the base meets the sides. Freeze.

Meanwhile, get going on your 'cheesecake' filling. Purée the avocado flesh, basil, the juice of three limes, 4 tablespoons of honey, the melted coconut oil and some Frank Sinatra at full speed until savagely smooth. I use my blender for this bit. Taste. If it needs more zing or kick, add another squeeze of lime juice to the mix. If you prefer more sweetness to rock your taste buds, then add an extra bit of honey. Spoon the filling over the frozen base and chill in the fridge for 1 hour. It will last for three days in the fridge like this.

Just before serving, slice a handful of fresh strawberries and scatter them over the top along with any stray basil leaves you find loitering in your kitchen.

FOR THE BASE:
1 ¹/₂ cups (180g) walnuts
6 Medjool or other sticky
  dates, stones removed
touch of sea salt flakes

FOR THE CREAMY CENTRE:
3 ripe avocados, stone and
  skin removed (240g)
25g packet of fresh basil,
  leaves only
juice of 3-4 limes
4-6 tablespoons raw honey
3 tablespoons unscented
  coconut oil, melted

FOR THE TOPPING:
1 punnet of fresh
  strawberries

Serves 8

MY WEDDING CAKE

XXXXXXXXXXXXX

It's hard to suppress the memory of making this cake at a demo and receiving a standing ovation. It was one of the most mortifying and confusing moments of my life. I must have missed a beat, because suddenly I was parading around the room holding it like the cup of Christ. I think they call this Jerusalem syndrome. Anyway, no one was harmed.

FOR THE BISCUIT BASE:
3 $1/2$ cups (420g) walnuts
12 Medjool dates, stones
  removed
$1/2$ teaspoon unrefined salt
squeeze of lemon juice

FOR THE FILLING:
4 $1/4$ cups (600g) raw
  unsalted cashews
1-1 $1/4$ cups (250-300ml) raw
  honey or light agave syrup
just over $3/4$ cup (190ml)
  melted coconut oil
flesh of 3 very ripe, juicy
  mangos
juice of 2-3 lemons
5 tablespoons freshly juiced
  ginger
4 teaspoons ground turmeric
edible flowers or rose
  petals, to decorate

Serves 60-70

First soak the cashews in a small bowl of water for at least 6 hours or overnight. Drain and discard the soaking liquid.

You'll need to oil three springform tins of ascending sizes: one 20cm tin, one 16cm tin and one 8cm tin. These are a special type of baking tin used to make cheesecakes and fancy tortes. You'll find them on Amazon. If you want a fourth larger tier, you'll need to do the entire recipe again and fill a single 25cm springform tin.

To make the base for all three tins, briefly pulse the listed ingredients together using a food processor. A blender will purée the ingredients, so it's essential to use a processor here. Stop the motor when the dough starts to clump together. Spread the nutty dough over the bottom of each of your three springform tins and place in the freezer to chill.

To make the filling, cream the softened cashews with the remaining filling ingredients (except the edible flowers) until smooth and glossy. This should take 2 minutes in a blender or food processor. Taste it and see whether you'd prefer more mango or ginger. Keep in mind that it will taste milder once frozen. Pour this creamy, luminous filling over your three bases and return to the freezer until set.

Allow the cakes to thaw for 5 minutes before removing them from their tins and stacking them on top of one another. Tickle with edible flowers. With a bit of luck, you'll only suffer from Stendahl syndrome.

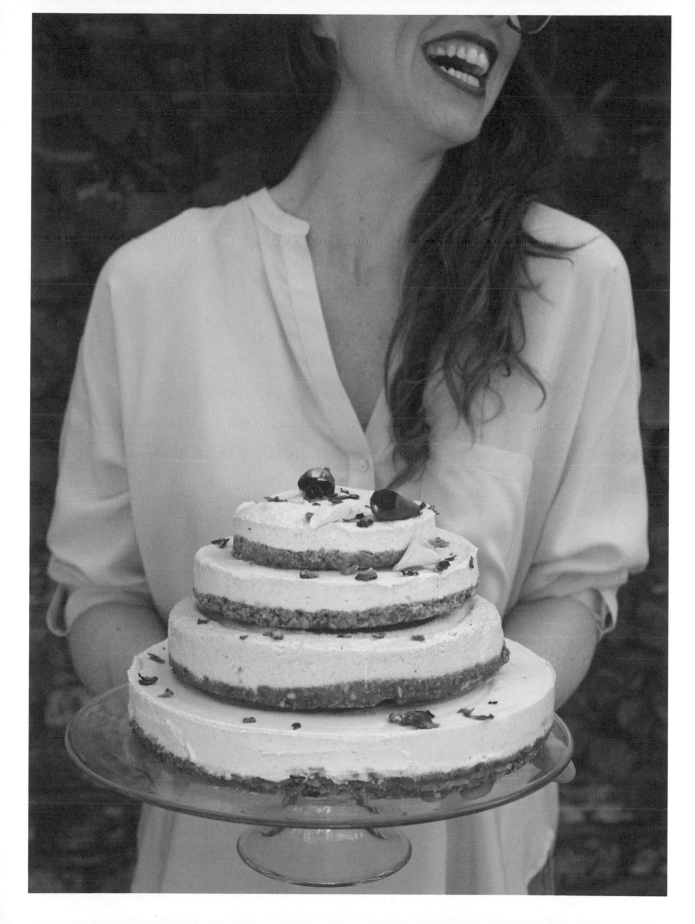

3

SAINTLY TREATS

TO SERVICE YOUR INNER DEVIL

BBQ KALE CRISPS

«»«»«»«»«»«»

Kale is unforgivably trendy. During London Fashion Week, kale ice pops were on the menu. I imagine one levitates with virtuousness after horsing into such a lolly. Every glossy magazine on the circuit seems to have a kale smoothie recipe by an equally glossy celebrity. I fear what's next. Cauliflower juice?

Truth is, kale is almost celestial. One leaf of this supergreen would have an acre of broccoli blushing. For a start, it has more antioxidants than the much-coveted blueberry. We like antioxidants for their special agent moves against the damaging free radicals loitering in our system. Think US Navy SEALs in the bloodstream. Gram for gram, kale has almost twice the vitamin C of an orange. This vitamin is hailed as our skin's greatest ally against ageing and dodgy office bugs. And kale's stock of iron is even higher than spinach. Hard luck, Popeye.

I'm still trying to make friends with this super veg. It's not easy, but here's one way it canters onto my dinner table.

500g curly kale
$\frac{1}{2}$ tablespoon extra virgin
  olive oil
$\frac{1}{2}$ teaspoon smoked paprika
$\frac{1}{2}$ teaspoon ground cumin
$\frac{1}{2}$ teaspoon sea salt flakes
$\frac{1}{4}$ teaspoon cayenne pepper

Serves 1-6 mouths

Crank up your oven to 200°C/180°C fan/400°F.

Tear the kale leaves from their tough stalks any old way – it doesn't matter – and put the leaves into a large bowl. Massage a little olive oil into the kale leaves. The less oil, the better, I find.

Roast the kale on your largest baking tray for 8-10 minutes, until crispy. If the leaves look a little crowded, give them space by using two roasting trays. They'll be crunchier as a result.

While the kale is doing its thing, add all the spices to an empty jam jar and shake it up. Remove your crispy kale chips from the oven and sprinkle over the spices. Taste. It's like magical fairy dust.

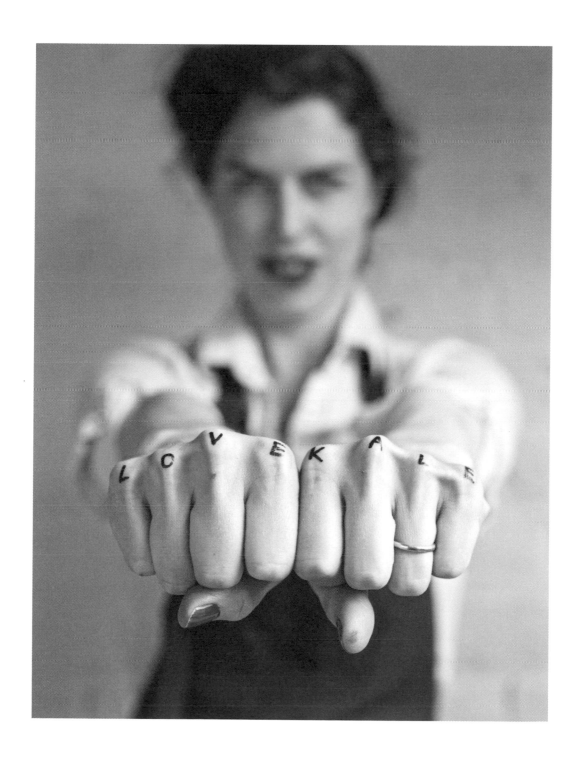

SAINTLY TREATS

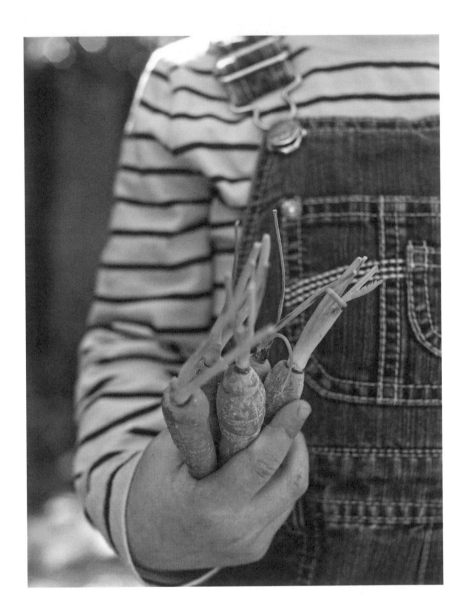

VEGETABLE CRISPS

《》《》《》《》《》《》

There's a touch of Derren Brown about them.

Unusually for a root vegetable, Jerusalem artichokes store inulin instead of starch. Inulin has been shown to feed the good bacteria in our gut. Score! Prebiotic crisps!

We're told that the levels at which a person can tolerate inulin can vary wildly. Some might get noisy with it, while others escape the gasworks. The litmus test is to try a few crisps the first night. If the air stays clear, go wild with a tray and your favourite box set.

Preheat the oven to 190°C/170°C fan/375°F.

Leaving the skin on, scrub any dirt or grit from the Jerusalem artichoke under fresh running water. Slice thinly and uniformly. If you have a fancy machine to do this, so much the better. Mandolines are good, but I prefer a Magimix food processor blade, designed to slice whole vegetables in less than two seconds.

Scatter the sliced arties over one or two roasting trays, depending on how many people you plan on serving. Parachute the sea salt flakes on top. Make sure each slice is spread out and isn't fraternising with another piece. They need to dry out in the oven, and they can't do that if they are love-bombing each other.

Bake in the oven for 12-20 minutes, depending on how thick the slices are. When the corner of a crisp starts to brown, take it out. Some might need to bake a bit longer.

Let them cool and crinkle on a wire rack for 10 minutes. Serve, keeping the secret to yourself. Please.

1 Jerusalem artichoke per person
a flurry of sea salt flakes

HOMEMADE COCONUT MILK YOGHURT

《》《》《》《》《》《》《》《》《》《》《》

If you have a dairy-free diet, then tasting coconut milk yoghurt is almost like a religious experience. Candida warriors will love it, as will your vegan pal and that hot Pilates instructor you've been dying to impress. Now you have an excuse to get his email address.

You can find blocks of coconut cream for less than a quid in your local Asian or ethnic grocer. At health food stores, expect to pay three times the price for organic varieties. No yoghurt-making machine required.

1 block (200g) coconut cream
 (aka creamed coconut, as
 in the photo)
1 $1/4$ cups (300ml) hot
 filtered water
1 teaspoon stevia Erylite
$1/4$ teaspoon or 2 capsules
 probiotic powder
$1/4$ vanilla bean, seeds
 scraped out, or pure
 vanilla powder

Makes 6-8 servings

Chop the coconut cream into small chunks, being careful not to include your fingers (the cream can be rock solid). Add to a blender or food processor along with the hot water and blend until smooth.

Leave to cool for 15 minutes before adding the stevia powder, probiotic powder and the vanilla seeds or powder. You could use the culture from a batch of CoYo or another natural yoghurt, but I find the probiotic powder to be more effective.

Pour into a scrupulously clean 750ml—1 litre Kilner jar and cover with kitchen paper or a clean muslin and an elastic band. I keep mine on the warm kitchen counter draped with muslin for 24-36 hours before tasting and refrigerating. You could of course leave yours in the boiler room or airing press to achieve similar results - you're aiming for 26°C. If it's particularly warm, 24 hours could be plenty of time to let the culture multiply.

Every 6 hours, or when I remember, I whisk it to ensure consistency and to prevent it from splitting. After a maximum of 36 hours, refrigerate and gobble within 10 days.

That's it!

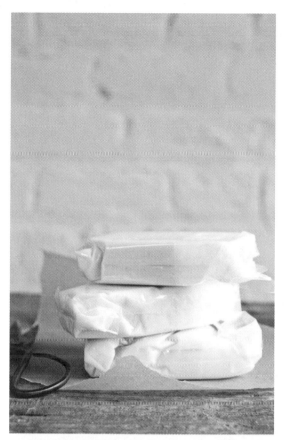

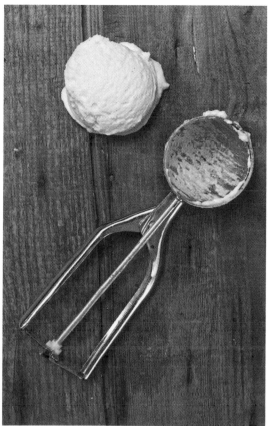

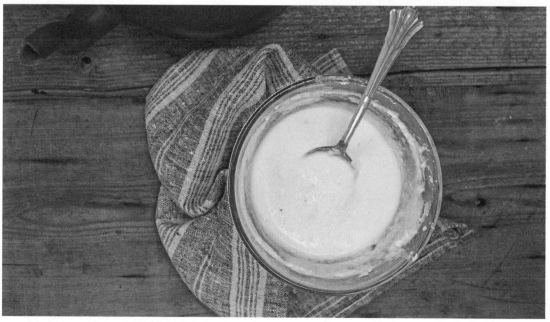

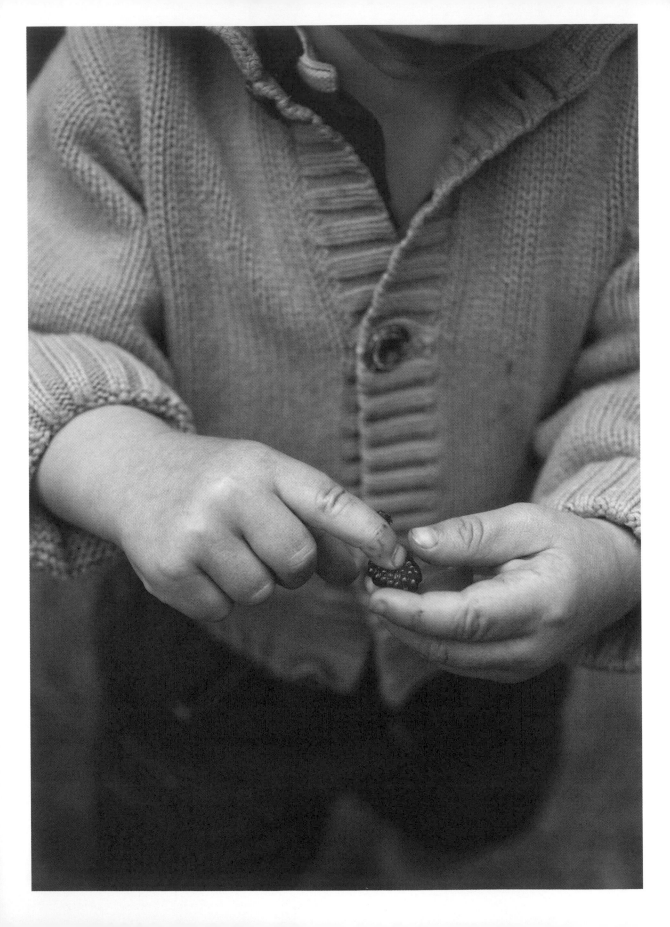

RASPBERRY JAM - THE HEALTHY KIND

≪≫≪≫≪≫≪≫≪≫≪≫≪≫≪≫≪≫≪≫≪≫≪≫≪≫

When you need to recharge your superhuman powers, try chia. These weensy seeds are members of the omega-3 plant squad. Why such excitement? Omega-3 is a good fat, the kind that nourishes your noggin, not your waistline.

Our brain cells are primarily composed of fat. So, too, are many of our neurons - think of an internal electricity grid that lights up our thoughts. There is strong scientific evidence linking good brain health with diets rich in omega-3s. I see little point in necking expensive pharma-bullets when I can be merrily tucking into this jam every morning.

Find black or white varieties of chia in your local health food store and on-trend grocers. Chia may initially seem expensive, but these tiny seeds actually swell to four times their volume as soon as liquid touches their orbit. Apart from being a tasty insurance policy against brain drain, chia seeds deliver a surprisingly generous dose of calcium and iron too. Great food for mama and bump.

To make the chia jam, pelt the thawed raspberries into a food processor with the licky-sticky dates, chia seeds and lime juice, or use a hand-held blender. Allow the chia seeds to thicken the jam for 30 minutes before using. I like to give it the odd stir every few minutes to prevent lumps.

Store in the fridge for up to one week. Tastes super on porridge and pancakes.

1 cup (150g) frozen
  raspberries, defrosted
3 dates, pre-soaked and
  stones removed
2 tablespoons chia seeds
squeeze of lime juice
  (optional)

Makes 10-12 single servings

TEFF, GINGER AND BLACK PEPPER COOKIES

《》《》《》《》《》《》《》《》《》《》《》《》《》《》《》《》

Cashews: are they fattening or not? In theory, yes. Nuts have rich stores of fat. In practice, no. Nuts are not 'fattening' unless you shovel titanic amounts into your diet. Given that they are naturally very filling, overeating would be very difficult. Even for Jay Rayner.

So here's the skinny. Many nuts, like the cashew, are rampant with monounsaturated fat. This is the heart-healthy fat associated with happier cholesterol readings. The British Medical Journal published research on seven foods, including nuts, which if consumed daily would reduce the risk of heart disease by 75%.

Given that heart disease is Ireland's number one killer, we would probably do well to solicit more raw, unsalted nuts into our diet. I love the idea of fighting disease with a fork.

1 cup (135g) unsalted cashew nuts

1 cup (90g) oat flakes

just under 1 cup (120g) teff flour

1 tablespoon milled chia seeds

3 teaspoons ground ginger

1/2 teaspoon baking powder

1/2 teaspoon sea salt flakes

several twists of the black pepper mill

2/3 cup (165ml) brown rice syrup

1/2 cup (125ml) melted extra virgin coconut oil

Makes 18-25 cookies

Preheat your oven to 180°C/160°C fan/350°F. Line two baking trays with parchment paper.

Finely grind the dry ingredients (everything except the syrup and melted oil) in a food processor until they resemble breadcrumbs. Try not to aim for a flour, as this would be too fine a consistency.

Add the brown rice syrup and melted coconut oil. Pulse again until a big dough ball forms in the bowl of your food processor. The key to these beauts is the brown rice syrup. Maple, honey or agave won't give these biscuits enough snap and chew. It's also worth making sure your salt is in flakes and not finely milled.

Pull off an apricot-sized piece of dough and roll it into a ball between your palms. Place on the lined baking tray and flatten each one with a spatula. I usually bake the cookies in batches or freeze half the cookie dough for another day.

Cook for 10-12 minutes, depending on their size - but no longer, promise me! - and remove from the oven before they turn a shade darker. Don't worry if they seem soft or undercooked - they will harden on the trays as they cool down.

Move over, Michael Fassbender. There's a new fixation in town.

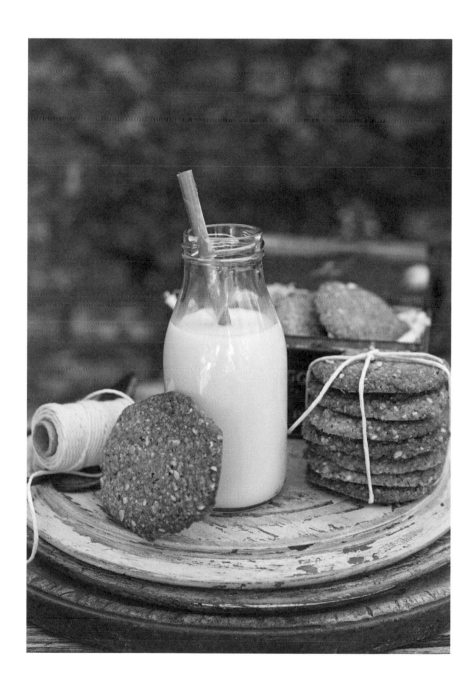

SAINTLY TREATS

ANTI-CHOLESTEROL COOKIES

《》《》《》《》《》《》《》《》《》《》

A high five for your ticker.

2 blackened, over-ripe
  bananas, mashed (about
  160g)
1 cup (90g) regular oats
  (not jumbo)
$1/2$ cup (45g) grated carrot
$1/3$ cup (50g) raisins
1 teaspoon baking powder
1 teaspoon ground cinnamon
some zest from $1/2$ unwaxed
  orange

Makes 16 cookies

Start by preheating your oven to 180°C/160°C
fan/350°F. You'll need two large baking trays
lined with parchment paper.

Beat all the ingredients together in a large bowl
with a fork and muscle.

Roll 1 tablespoon of the dough into a ball
between your palms like Play-Doh, then gently
flatten the top and bottom. Arrange on the lined
baking trays. They won't spread while cooking, so
you can arrange them quite closely.

Cook for 12 minutes or a little longer if the
cookies are big, until firm enough to hold without
collapsing. Let them cool for 30 minutes on a
wire rack before packing into pockets and lunch
boxes.

AMERICAN PEANUT BUTTER COOKIES

《》《》《》《》《》《》《》《》《》《》《》《》《》

Lenny Kravitz, on the lips.

Preheat the oven to 180°C/160°C fan/350°F. Line two baking trays with parchment paper.

Blend all the ingredients together in a large bowl with a fork. Roll into little ping pong-sized balls and place on the lined trays. They will flatten naturally when the heat hits them.

Bake for 10-12 minutes, before they turn brown or crisp. Don't panic if they appear soft - you're on the right track because they harden once cooled.

Resist the temptation to wolf them hot from the oven. I'm still nursing my sore tongue.

$^3/_4$ cup (200g) smooth or crunchy peanut butter
$^3/_4$ cup (100g) coconut sugar or $^1/_2$ cup (100g) stevia Erylite
4 tablespoons milled chia seeds (optional)
1 teaspoon baking powder
1 egg

Makes 16-20 cookies

YOUR HEALTH IS AN INVESTMENT, NOT AN EXPENSE.

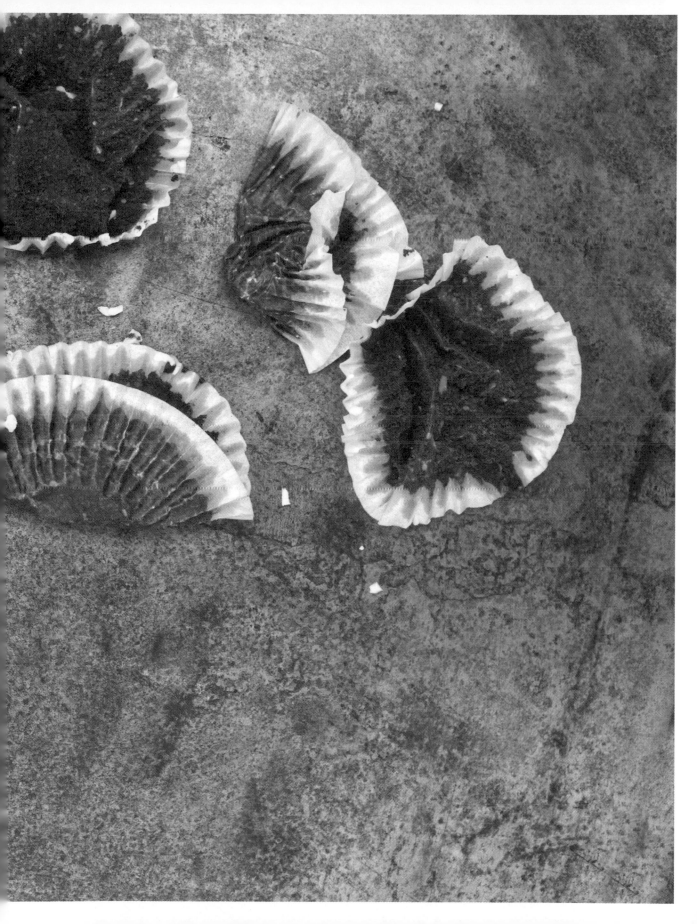

CAMU CAMU COOKIES

≪≫≪≫≪≫≪≫≪≫≪≫

Camu camu is the latest health industry pom-pom. This Amazonian fruit has explosive amounts of vitamin C - more than a wheelbarrow of oranges and lemons. Sounds like a potent anti-ageing ally to have.

2 cups (200g) ground almonds
$1/2$ cup (125ml) extra virgin
  coconut oil, melted
$1/3$ cup (80ml) maple syrup,
  raw honey or coconut
  nectar
1 tablespoon camu camu
  powder
1 teaspoon ground turmeric
1 teaspoon ground ginger
generous pinch of sea salt
  flakes

Makes 20 cookies

These cookies don't need to be baked. Using a fork, mix everything together in a cold bowl. Transfer the dough between two large sheets of non-stick baking parchment. Roll out like pastry until it's 1cm thick. Freeze on a flat surface for 20 minutes.

Retrieve the firm dough from the freezer and cut into cookie shapes. I use regular cookie cutters, but you could also use a pizza slicer to cut out squares. I tip them into a ziplock bag while they are still nicely frozen.

Return the cookies to the freezer for storage, ready to plunder when the need arises. These cookies don't even need to be defrosted - you can eat them straight away. Groovy, huh?

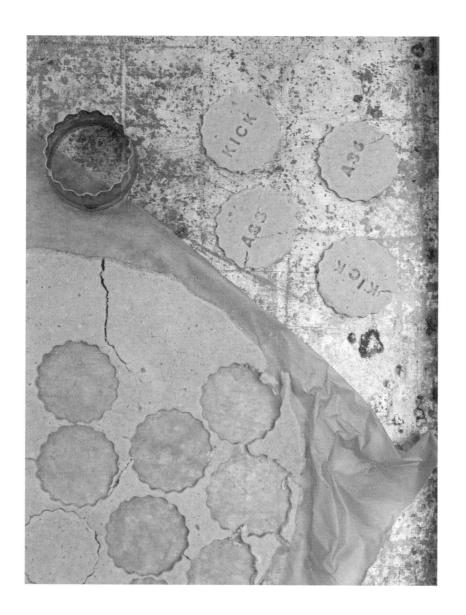

SAINTLY TREATS

LEONARD COHEN FLAPJACKS

《》《》《》《》《》《》《》《》《》《》

If you think you need to bridle your jaw around chocolate, it might be worth scrolling through your iPod. Research shows that sad music encourages us to overeat. Participants in a recent trial were split into two groups: one exposed to upbeat ballet, the other to the sombre tones of Prokofiev (it was a toss-up between Prokofiev and Leonard Cohen). Then both groups were shown how to obtain chocolate buttons by pressing a keyboard linked to a dispenser. Those exposed to Prokofiev clicked their computers almost three times more than those who listened to the ballet.

We hardly need science to solve this phenomenon. Some of us are programmed to regulate our moods with industrial quantities of chocolate. It's written in our constitution, innit? Nevertheless, it did get me dissecting my lists on Spotify with the nervous expertise of a first-grade surgeon employing a scalpel.

So I got thinking. What if you could turn your sugar calling into a nutritional slam-dunk? That's when I came up with this beaut, with hidden vats of quinoa. He and I have been best friends ever since.

²/₃ cup (160ml) extra virgin
  coconut oil
¹/₃ cup (80ml) honey (not
  maple syrup)
1 teaspoon ground cinnamon
1 teaspoon vanilla extract
8 Medjool dates or pre-
  soaked regular dates,
  stones removed
3 cups (270g) regular oat
  flakes (not jumbo)
³/₄ cup (90g) quinoa flour
¹/₃ cup (50g) pumpkin seeds,
  chopped
1 ripe banana, mashed
handful of chocolate chips
  (optional)
¹/₂ teaspoon sea salt flakes

Makes 30 flapjacks

A few snoresome but important housekeeping notes: use extra virgin coconut oil rather than regular or odourless oil. Something gross happens to the latter. A palmful of chocolate chips is advised for the fuss artist in the family. Quinoa flour can be replaced with ground almonds if you don't dig this groovy grain. And standard oats work much better than jumbo ones. Confused? Me too. But who cares about the science when they taste so freakishly good?

Preheat the oven to 170°C/150°C fan/340°F. Line a 30cm x 20cm baking tin (the size of an A4 page) with non-stick baking parchment. I swear by the If You Care brand and find most others to be imposters.

Start by gently warming the coconut oil and honey in a deep, large saucepan over a low heat until they look happily ensconced. Add the cinnamon and vanilla.

Meanwhile, roughly chop the dates and toss them into the syrupy mix before adding the remaining ingredients. Mix thoroughly.

Press into your prepared tin and bake for 30 minutes, before the oats have a chance to turn brown. Remove from the oven and allow to cool completely in the tin before attempting to hack off a few slices. I store mine in the fridge to keep them from crumbling, but they will survive perfectly in children's lunch boxes.

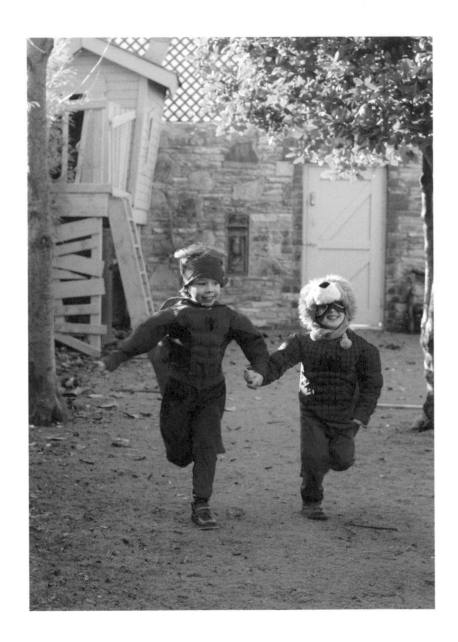

SUPERHERO TIFFIN

《》《》《》《》《》《》

Traditional tiffin is home to broken biscuits, white sugar, cheap fat, golden syrup, chocolate and undisputed pleasure. It's a childhood favourite among millions, including me.

This version of tiffin brings incalculable happiness to my home: fudgy, chewy chunks of 'chocolatey' fruit 'n' nut with no refined muck to compromise your health.

Carob isn't actually chocolate. It's closer to mild coffee and vanilla beans. People confuse its colour with that of cocoa. Carob is a member of the pea family and offers powerful antioxidants like quercetin and protective catechins as well as modest amounts of vitamins A, D, B, iron, calcium and magnesium. Ooh argh.

Isn't it so cool to find a snack you love that loves you back?

Find a small container that's the size of your hand. It needs to be as deep as half your hand. A small lunch box is perfect. Line with one sheet of cling film.

With a fork and muscle, beat the tahini, syrup, carob powder, vanilla extract and a pinch of sea salt together. Thoroughly. Stir through the raisins, walnuts, cacao nibs (if using) and the odd red goji berry. Beat in the coconut oil.

Quickly transfer to your lined container and press a few goji berries on the top before placing in the freezer to set. Once set, remove from the container, wrap in baking parchment, return to the freezer and raid at will.

1 cup (250ml) best-quality light or dark tahini
6–8 tablespoons maple, date or carob syrup
1 tablespoon carob powder
$\frac{1}{2}$ teaspoon real vanilla extract
sprinkle of sea salt flakes
handful of raisins
handful of walnuts
handful of raw cacao nibs (optional)
handful of goji berries
2 tablespoons extra virgin coconut oil, melted

Makes 20-30 portions

HONUTS - THE HEALTHY DONUT

≪≫≪≫≪≫≪≫≪≫≪≫≪≫≪≫≪≫≪≫

This recipe is based on the classic donut from Babycakes NYC, a gluten-free bakery that FedExes donuts across the country to breathless celebs. I know it seems like an intemperate amount of ingredients to purchase, but you'll be guaranteed year-round honuts and happiness. Admittedly, these honuts flirt with their own mortality after 6 hours. Best to eat them straight away, like at a picnic, DVD night or children's party.

For more on jaggery as a choice of sweetener, see page 12.

³/₄ cup (100g) coconut sugar, rapadura or jaggery
³/₄ cup (90g) brown rice flour and/or sorghum flour
¹/₂ cup (80g) potato flour
¹/₃ cup (40g) chickpea flour
4 tablespoons arrowroot
1 tablespoon ground cinnamon
2 teaspoons baking powder
¹/₂ teaspoon xanthan gum
pinch of sea salt flakes
just under ³/₄ cup (160ml) hot water
just over ¹/₃ cup (90ml) coconut oil, melted
6 tablespoons apple purée
1 teaspoon vanilla powder or extract

Makes 10-12 donuts

We are going to bake these donuts instead of deep-frying the bejaysus out of them, so start by preheating your oven to 180°C/160°C fan/350°F.

Using some of your melted coconut oil, brush two six-mould donut trays and set aside. I only have one donut tray, so I end up doing two batches, which works just fine.

Spin all the dry ingredients together in a blender or food processor. Now add the wet ingredients: your hot water, melted coconut oil, apple purée and vanilla. Blitz until sumptuous and smooth.

Drop spoonfuls of batter into each donut mould. Use the end of your spoon handle to drag the batter around the ring.

Bake for 20-22 minutes. Let them cool in the mould for 5 minutes before releasing with a silicone knife.

Eat them hot, to hit your serotonin and your toes. I dipped these into a sneaky icing made with cacao butter, maple syrup and beetroot powder.

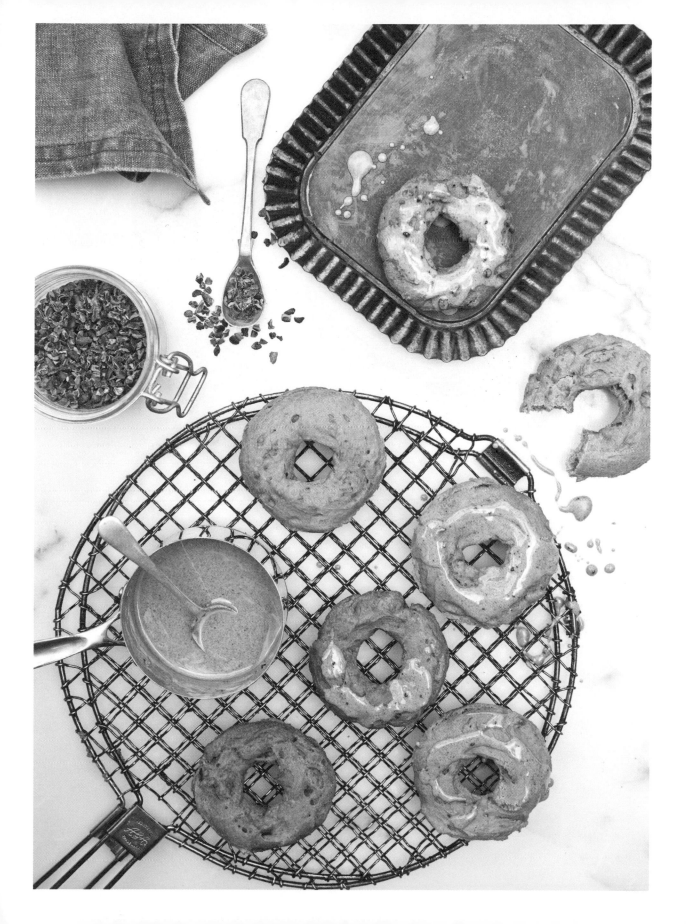

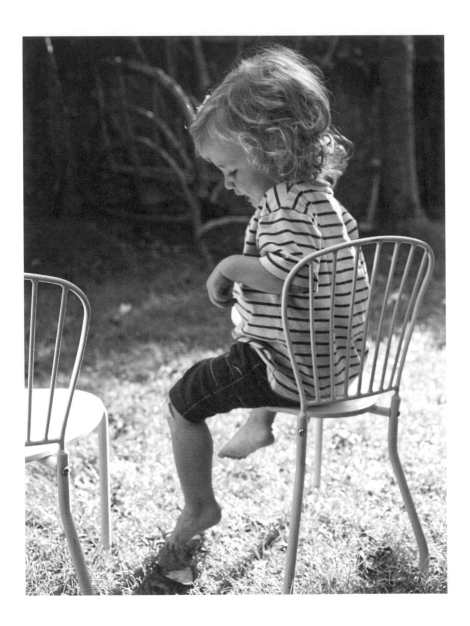

CHIA BREAKFAST PUD WITH PASSION FRUIT AND SEA SALT

《》«》《》«》«》«》«》«》《》«》«》《》«》«》«》《》«》«》《》«》«》«》《》«》«》

Can bananas cure dementia? No, but evidence suggests they can arm our brain with an armada of essential nutrients to get our neurotransmitters breakdancing for longer. 'In every great production, there are hundreds of people behind the scenes that support the main players,' writes Dr Hyla Cass, professor of psychiatry. 'The same is true with your brain. These are the vitamins and minerals. They help build and rebuild the brain and nervous system, and keep everything running smoothly. They are your brain's best friends.'

Of particular interest to Dr Cass are the B group vitamins. A deficiency in B6, she notes, raises our risk of developing depression and can antagonise mental health problems. B6 plays a critical role in the production of serotonin, the feel-good hormone in our body. No serotonin, no samba. The good news? B6 is found in bananas, chickpeas, beans, nuts and many whole grains. These are your new BFs.

Patrick Holford stresses the importance of 'smart fats' that fertilise the brain. Think sardines, mackerel, salmon, herring, chia, hempseed and flax. These superfoods all contain essential fatty acids that go on to manufacture top-class brain cells and other brain-related nomenclature. Mamasita likes the sound of that, especially as the foods he lists are so stonking delicious. To date, scientific literature on the consumption of essential fatty acids overwhelmingly suggests that subjects (that's you and me) experience a notable increase in mental clarity and agility.

The hallmark of a brainbox? This chia and banana pudding.

Stir the mashed banana, hemp milk, chia seeds and sea salt in a tall pint glass. Leave for 30 minutes or overnight in the fridge. I like to stir the pudding several times in the first 10 minutes to prevent globby hunks from forming.

When the chia seeds have swelled and absorbed all the yumminess, scoop out the flesh from the passion fruits to crown each serving. Wickedly good with a lick of honey or coconut nectar.

Leftovers will last for up to three days in the fridge.

1 banana, mashed
just under 1 1/2 cups (350ml) plant-based milk, like hemp (page 10)
5 tablespoons milled or whole chia seeds
pinch of sea salt flakes
3 passion fruits
raw honey or coconut nectar

Makes 3-4 servings

APPLE AND WINTER SQUASH CRUMBLE

《》《》《》《》《》《》《》《》《》《》《》《》

Butternut is a type of squash as well as a euphemism for Michelin-starred chefs. And Mary Berry. However, the butternut is not a nut at all. But by golly, does it taste sweet and buttery.

This vegetable is carbalicious and full of stonking nutrients such as beta-carotene and potassium. One cup of butternut is likely to give you more than twice the amount of potassium than your average supplement, and rings in at a heavy 750µg of vitamin A. We love potassium to help keep our blood pressure dandy - too much sodium pushes blood pressure up, while potassium helps coax levels back down. Nifty, huh?

FOR THE FILLING:
$^1/_3$ of a butternut squash
  (300g)
1 tablespoon extra virgin
  coconut oil or ghee
roughly $^1/_2$ cup (100g) sticky
  dried prunes, chopped
flurry of ground cinnamon
flurry of ground ginger
just under 2 $^1/_2$ cups (600ml)
  apple purée

FOR THE CRUMBLE:
1 $^1/_2$ cups (135g) oat flakes
1 cup (135g) pumpkin seeds
4-5 tablespoons coconut
  nectar or maple syrup
4 tablespoons extra virgin
  coconut oil or ghee
generous pinch of sea salt
  flakes

Greek yoghurt or coconut
  milk yoghurt (page 130),
  to serve

Serves 10

Preheat the oven to 180°C/160°C fan/350°F.

To prep the filling, peel the butternut using a vegetable peeler. Scoop out the seeds, then chop some of the flesh into mouth-sized pieces. You'll only be using a third of a butternut (you just need 300g for the recipe), so you could make a great soup with the remainder. Tumble the chopped butternut onto a roasting tray, dot with the coconut oil or ghee and bake for 30 minutes, until caramelised and tender.

Get going on your topping. Briefly blitz all the crumble ingredients together for a few seconds in a food processor (not a blender).

Take the tray of yumminess out of the oven, transfer the squash to a casserole dish and scatter over the chopped prunes and spices. Mix through the apple purée. Now it's ready to cover with the crumble and bake for 20-30 minutes, being watchful that the top doesn't brown and turn bitter.

Serve as a wholesome breakfast with great clouds of Greek or coconut milk yoghurt. Will last all week in the fridge.

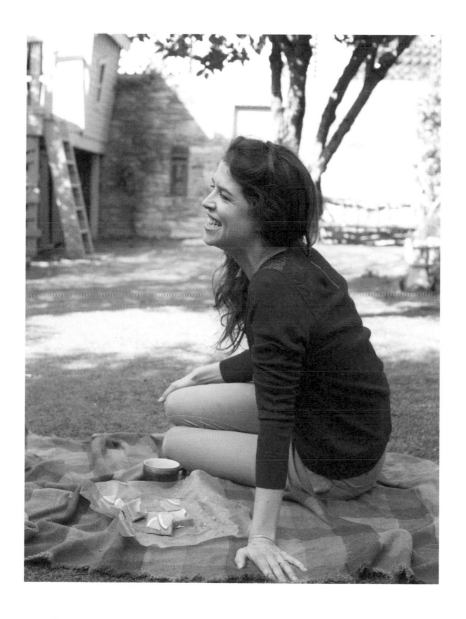

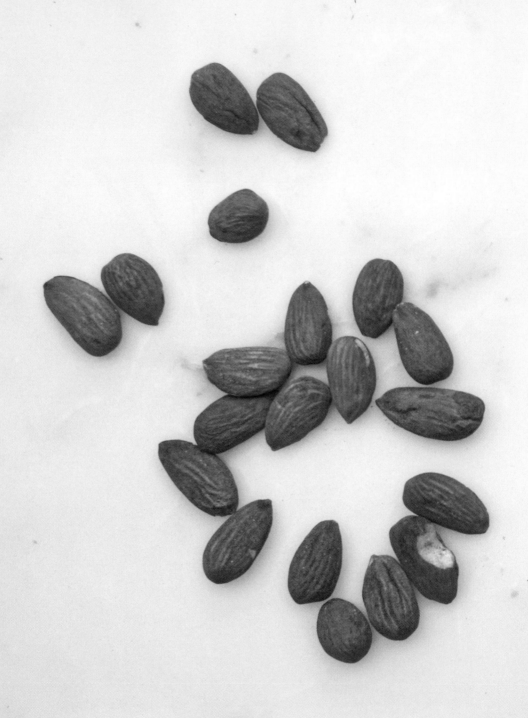

EATING POORLY WILL SHORT-CIRCUIT YOUR SYSTEM.

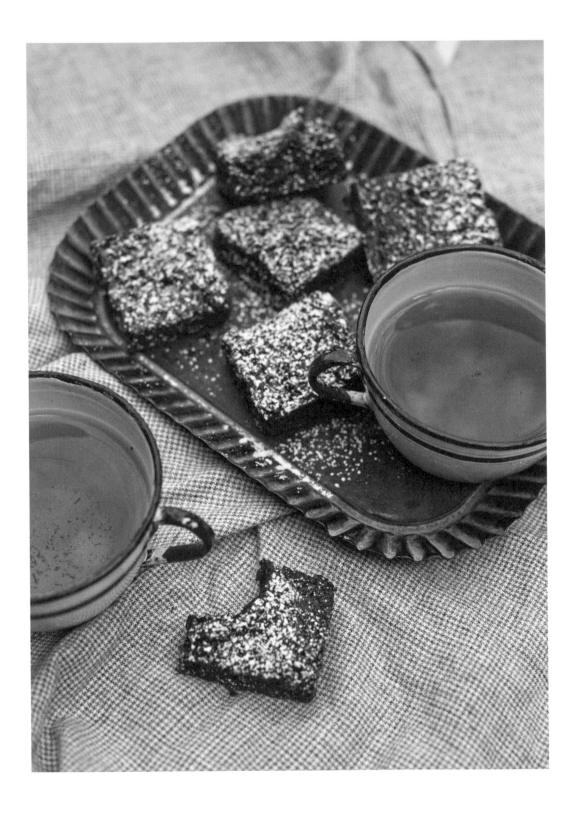

SECRET AGENT GINGERBREAD

《》《》《》《》《》《》《》《》《》

For a sugar, blackstrap molasses is a surprisingly good source of iron and is particularly useful for vegetarians or moody teens. Without sufficient iron, our bodies struggle to make haemoglobin. This is the stuff that helps transport oxygen around our system. No oxygen, no mojo. Busted. Sound familiar, ladies? That's because iron deficiency is more common in women than in men.

One tablespoon of blackstrap molasses also shoots us with 15% of our recommended calcium intake, making honey warble with envy. Breathless yet? And get this - chia is another fabulous plant source of calcium, so I've lobbed both ingredients into this gingerbread and kissed it with rum. Milled chia costs more than flour, but has an entire fleet of nutrients, like calcium, iron, omega-3, magnesium and protective plant lignans, to get your blood partying.

This gingerbread ain't sweet, not even slightly. Good to file under savoury. I sprinkle my gingerbread with probiotic powder. It looks like icing sugar to the kids and tastes nearly as sweet too.

Preheat the oven to 170°C/150°C fan/340°F. Instead of baking this gingerbread in a loaf pan, I use a 20cm x 20cm square brownie tin. This is because you need the dough to be as flat as possible. Line with parchment paper.

Stir all the dry ingredients together in a large bowl so that you don't get clumps of baking powder or ground ginger in any one spot.

Using a separate bowl, whisk the mashed banana with the ground chia seeds, apple juice or plant milk, molasses, melted fat, rum (if using) and vinegar. Pour into the dry ingredients and whip it into submission. This will take 5-6 minutes. Alternatively, you can throw everything into a blender or food processor - the texture will be smoother. Scrape the batter into your lined brownie tin and rake the top with a fork.

Bake for 35-40 minutes to get a sticky, dense gingerbread. Don't be disappointed if it looks flat. Just wait until you taste it! Allow to cool a little before cutting into bite-sized squares and using as currency. Can be stored for a week in parchment paper.

THE DRY INGREDIENTS:
2 cups (200g) ground almonds
3 tablespoons ground ginger
1 tablespoon carob powder
 (for colour)
1 teaspoon baking powder
1 teaspoon ground cinnamon
pinch of ground nutmeg
pinch of sea salt flakes

THE WET INGREDIENTS:
1 large banana, mashed
 (about 80g)
$^1/_2$ cup (45g) milled chia
 seeds
$^1/_2$ cup (125ml) apple juice
 or plant milk
5 tablespoons blackstrap
 molasses
4 tablespoons melted coconut
 oil or ghee
1 teaspoon rum (optional)
1 teaspoon apple cider
 vinegar or freshly
 squeezed lemon juice

Makes 10-16 portions

ANTI-AGEING CHOCOLATE MOUSSE

≪≫≪≫≪≫≪≫≪≫≪≫≪≫≪≫≪≫≪≫

What happens as we age? We're not as quick to solve problems, while multitasking can seem as tortuous as understanding string theory. That's because our cognitive ability begins to decrease. We're inclined to get more stressed and snappy as our concentration levels lapse. Our bones thin. Our arteries narrow. Our bodies creak. Our broad mind and narrow waist begin to change places. Gah!

Is ageing inescapable? No, but we can certainly change the speed at which we age. Surely that's a thrilling concept?

New genetic research claims that human beings may one day have a lifespan of 400 years. Embryologist Lewis Wolpert says this is because normal genes do not promote ageing, and no one dies of the condition 'old age'. Rather, complications arise that make recovery that bit trickier in an increasingly frail body. But what if we could optimise our well-being? Nurture our vitality? Offer stronger, robust genes to generations to come?

So are we programmed to age? Or is it that our body's repair mechanism just packs up? This difference could be crucial to genetic scientists. And, of course, to you.

How can we improve our chances of having a healthy old age? If we nourish our cells, our cells will nourish us. Let me help you do exactly that.

Play around with flavours: fresh ginger, chai spices, matcha green tea powder, lavender, baobab, lúcuma, acai, mandarin oil, black pepper and sea salt. Give it your signature.

2 ripe avocados, flesh only
6 tablespoons cacao powder
4 tablespoons maple syrup or coconut nectar
3 tablespoons nut butter
2-3 teaspoons tamari or coconut aminos
1/2 teaspoon real vanilla extract (optional)
seeds from 1/4 pomegranate, to decorate
coconut pouring cream, to serve

Serves 4

Pulse all the ingredients (except the pomegranate seeds and coconut pouring cream) together with a hand-held blender. It's best chilled for 30 minutes before wolfing, but excitement may over-ride your sensibilities. No shame in that.

Dish the mousse into glass tumblers and top with the antioxidant-rich pomegranate seeds. Really fabulous served with coconut pouring cream - just use coconut milk in place of the creamed coconut in the recipe for homemade coconut milk yoghurt on page 130.

This mousse is a great recipe to make ahead of time for a supper party, even up to three days in advance, as long as no one else knows where it's stored. You can also use it as a sneaky breakfast straight from the fridge. Not so great as a face mask.

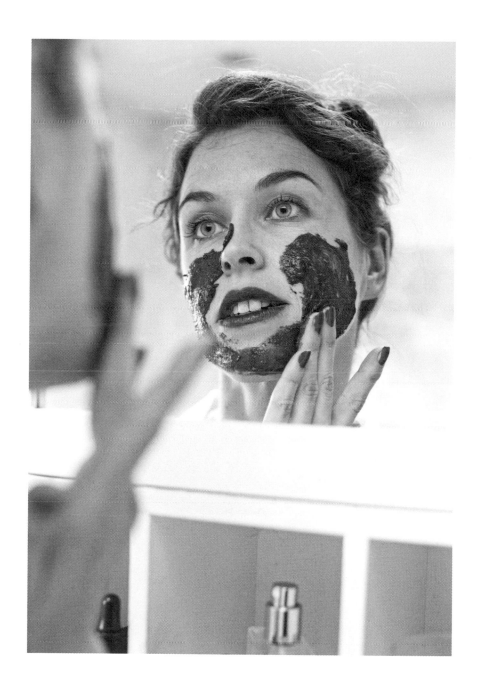

SAINTLY TREATS

CHOCOLATE SEED SOLDIERS

《》《》《》《》《》《》《》《》《》《》

These seed soldiers are excellent allies in the war against afternoon slumps. Practically humming with energy, they will deliver a cargo of essential minerals to service your mojo alongside battery-boosting B vitamins.

Goji berries are total beauts. Rich in iron, protein, super carotenoids and vitamins C, E and A (seriously!), these dainty berries are patently potent. We love carotenoids and vitamins C and E for their immune-pumping qualities. Think of these vitamins as ammo against the sniffles and dodgy office viruses. A deficiency in these vitamins can also make our skin look as dull as a tombstone. This is why the Chinese like to call goji berries 'red diamonds' - a girl's best friend.

Scientific evidence consistently proves that eating well is good for body and mind. Eating poorly will short-circuit your system. Once you taste these, I promise you'll never cavort with the office vending machine again. Try sneaking a tray into the staff fridge. They'll help extend deadlines.

1 cup (140g) pitted dates, chopped
1 cup (120g) milled sunflower and pumpkin seeds
¹/₂ cup (140g) cashew nut butter
¹/₂ cup (75g) raisins
¹/₂ cup (65g) coconut flour
¹/₂ cup (125ml) maple syrup (not honey)
3 tablespoons raw cacao nibs
2 tablespoons goji berries, plus extra to decorate
up to 1 tablespoon tamari or raw coconut aminos
130g 75% dark chocolate

Makes 20 generous portions

In a food processor (a simple fork and a temper will also work), combine everything except the dark chocolate and decorative gojies.

Spread it out over a parchment-lined shallow tin. The perfect size tin is a 20cm x 25cm rectangular one, a little larger than the traditional 20cm x 20cm square brownie tin. I place another piece of parchment paper on top of the base mixture, pressing down firmly with my fingers. Once the base is smooth, you can ditch the top piece of parchment. Chill in the fridge.

Meanwhile, slowly melt the chocolate in a bain-marie. This is basically a pot of simmering water, 2.5cm in depth, with a heatproof bowl sitting on top where a lid might otherwise have gone. The contents of the bowl will gently melt from the steam of the water underneath. The trick is not to let the water boil or let the bottom of the bowl touch the water underneath.

Smother the chilled base in melted chocolate and parachute a couple of goji berries on top for colour. Refrigerate overnight. I doubt you'll need an alarm clock to wake you up in the morning.

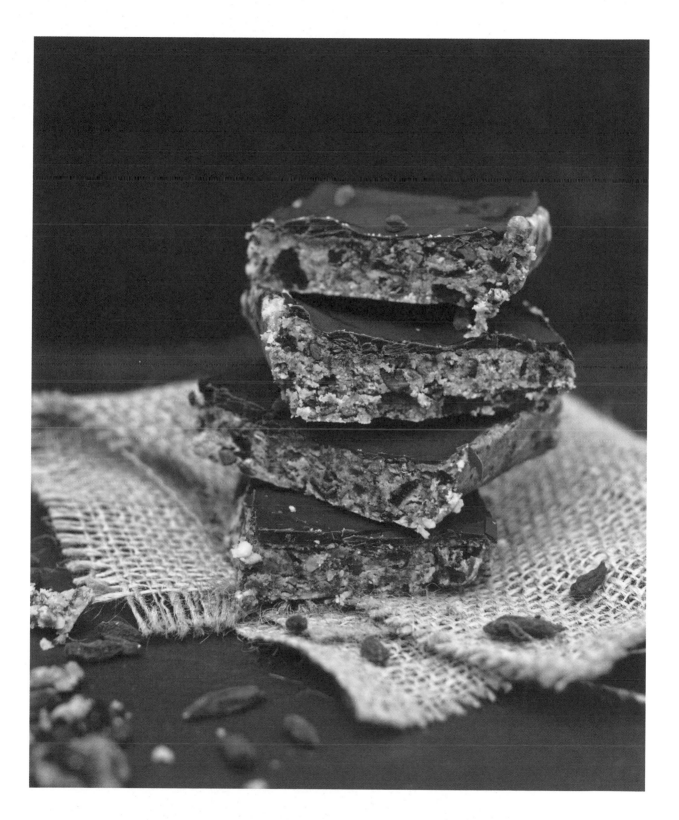

SAINTLY TREATS

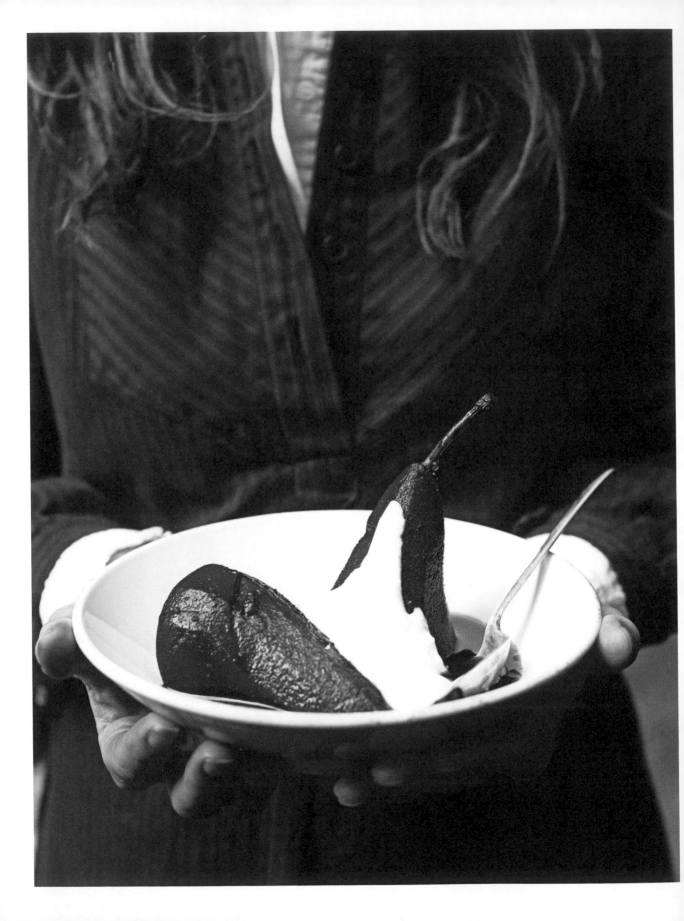

POACHED PEARS WITH STAR ANISE

《》《》《》《》《》《》《》《》《》《》《》《》《》

Promises to leave an indelible dance on your tongue.

Bring the red wine, orange juice and your chosen syrup to a rolling boil in a saucepan. Add the cloves, cinnamon stick and star anise. Let it simmer for 5 minutes while you peel the pears. I like to leave the stem intact and slice the bottom of the pears to create a flat arse. Gently place the peeled pears in your poaching liquid, cover the pan and simmer for 20-25 minutes, until tender. It's useful to turn the pears every so often to ensure they poach evenly.

Remove the saucepan from the heat, uncover and delicately take the pears out. Now reduce the poaching liquid over a medium-high heat for 25 minutes, until the liquid is more viscous and slightly syrupy.

Chill in the fridge for a few days or serve the pears straight away on individual plates, drizzled with the licky-sticky poaching liquid. (You could cut large pears in half to serve eight.) A dollop of coconut milk yoghurt takes the dish up an octave.

just over 1 ³/₄ cups (450ml) red wine
juice of 1 orange
3 tablespoons maple or brown rice syrup
2 whole cloves
1 cinnamon stick
1 star anise
4 firm, ripe pears
coconut milk yoghurt (page 130) or Greek yoghurt, to serve

Serves 4-8

POMEGRANATE HALVA

《》《》《》《》《》《》

Good enough to make a devout friar feel like John Travolta. Buying 36 individual portions of halva will cost you the same price as an inkjet printer. My version costs way less than a cartridge.
Pomegranate halva is as close as you'll come to an orgasm with your clothes on.

3 tablespoons extra virgin coconut oil
up to $^1/_2$ cup (125ml) maple syrup, coconut nectar, agave or raw honey
1 teaspoon vanilla extract
pinch of sea salt flakes
340g light tahini
4 tablespoons pomegranate seeds
2-3 tablespoons runny raw honey

Makes 36 portions

On a very timid heat, gently melt the coconut oil in a small saucepan. Let your preferred choice of syrup, the vanilla and a pinch of salt join the party. With a fork, beat through the tahini and pomegranate seeds. Keep back some ruby red seeds to tickle the top.

Scrape half the mixture into a small rectangular container lined with cling film. Dribble some runny honey over it and scrape the remaining mixture over it. Prod it with a fork and give it a swirl to move the honey about without incorporating it into the tahini. These will taste like caramel swirls. Decorate with some more pom seeds.

Freeze for 4 hours. Just like ice cream, the halva must be stored in the freezer or else it will melt into a holy mess. Slice big cubes from it and marvel at its virtuous decadence.

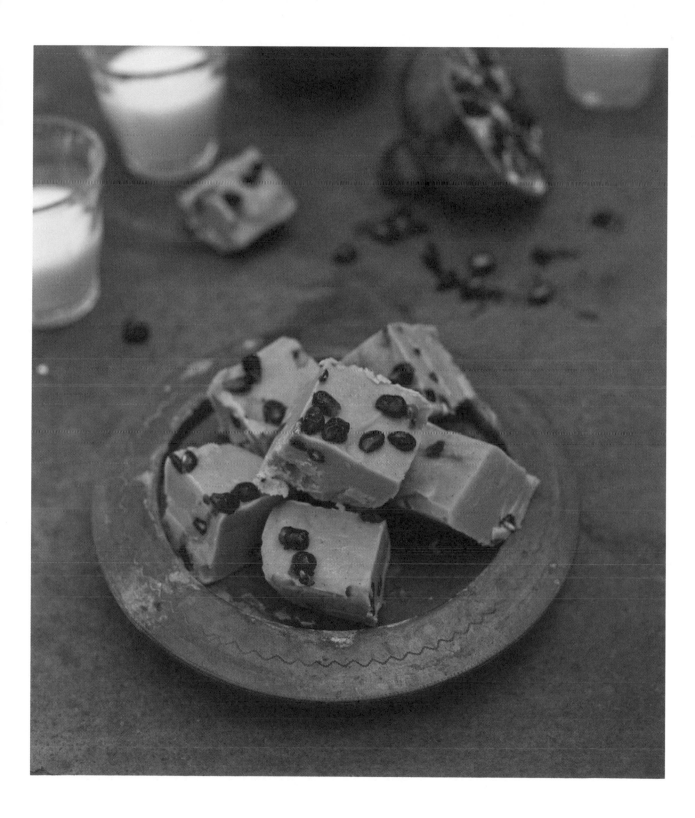

SAINTLY TREATS

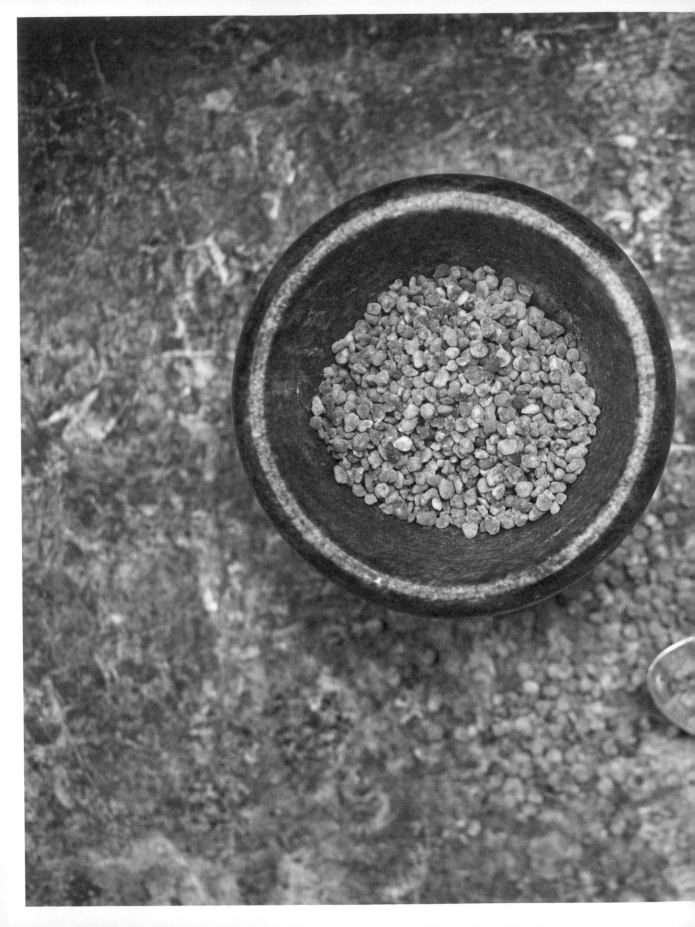

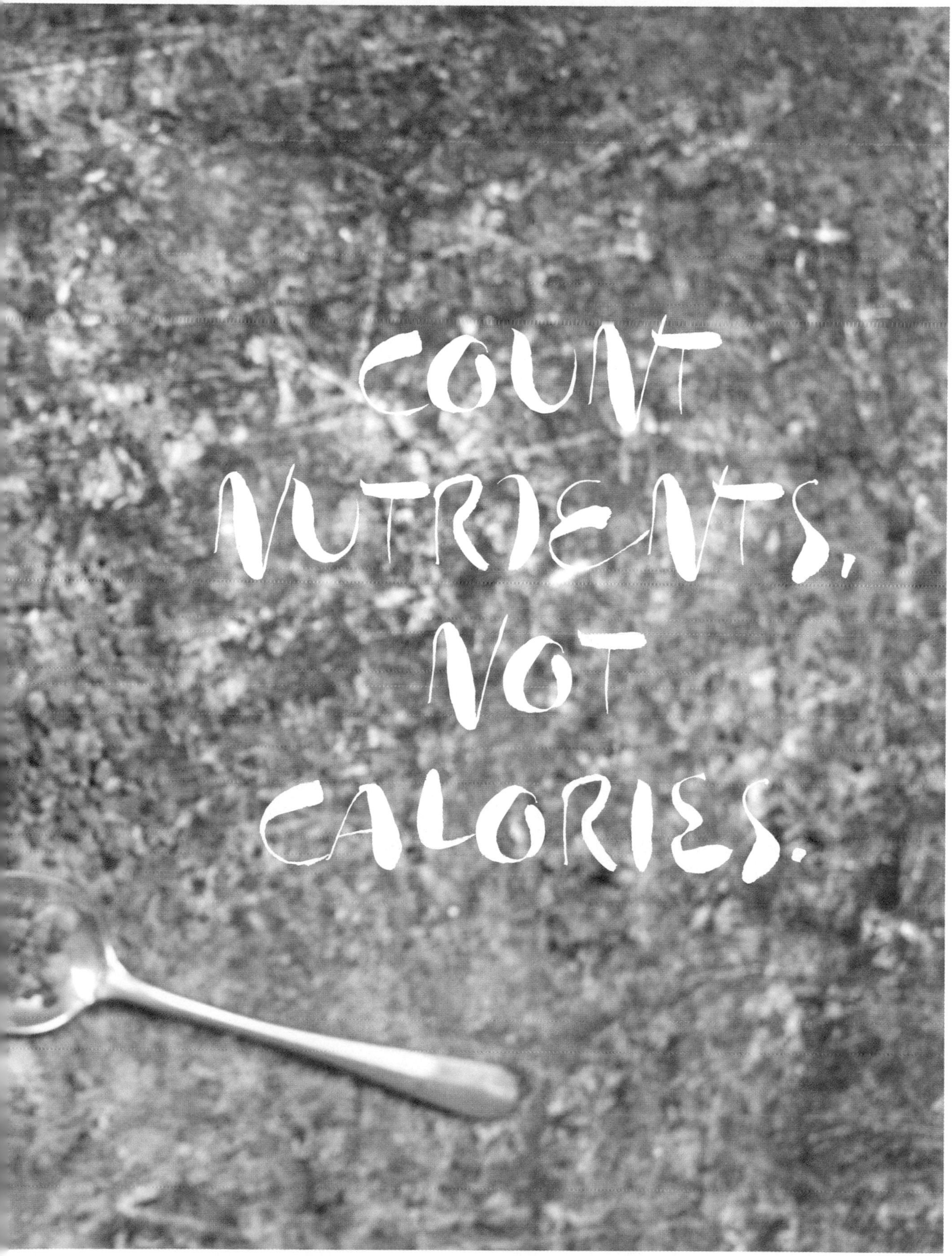
COUNT
NUTRIENTS,
NOT
CALORIES.

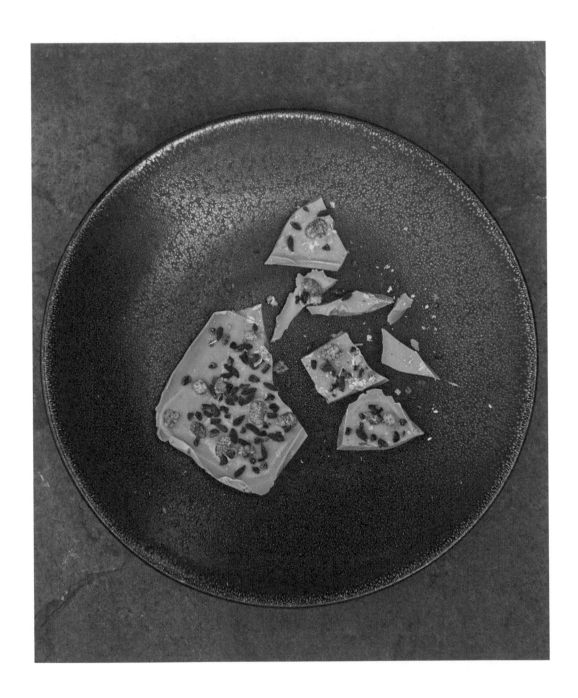

WHITE CHOCOLATE BARK WITH A TOUCH OF SEA SALT

«»«»«»«»«»«»«»«»«»«»«»«»«»«»«»«»«»«»

Release your inner Mary Poppins.

First line a large loaf tin with parchment paper or cling film.

Melt the raw cacao butter in a bain-marie. This is basically a pot of simmering water, 2.5cm in depth, with a heatproof bowl sitting on top where a lid might otherwise have gone. The contents of the bowl will gently melt from the steam of the water underneath. The trick is not to let the water violently boil or let the bottom of the bowl touch the water underneath.

Warm up your blender with hot water. Pour out the water, then blitz the melted cacao butter with your lúcuma and quickly pour into the lined loaf tin. Freeze immediately for a maximum of 2 minutes (exclamation mark!). Do not leave unattended because you'll miss the opportunity to add the real jazz.

Take the tin out of the freezer and parachute the remaining ingredients on top before it sets completely. Return to the freezer for another 10-15 minutes. Once the bark is solid, store it in the fridge.

When you need to serve, drop the bark onto a wooden chopping board and watch it shatter into fabulous shards. Amen.

100g solid cacao butter
3 tablespoons lúcuma powder
pinch of goji berries
pinch of dried mulberries
pinch of cacao nibs
pinch of sea salt flakes

Makes 8 portions

THAT LEMON CURD

≪≫≪≫≪≫≪≫≪≫

Here are two things you should know about egg yolks that you won't read on the side of an egg box. Firstly, these little golden treasures contain military amounts of phospholipids called choline and inositol. Phospholipids have several important functions in our bodies, most notably for the proper breakdown of fats in our diet. Delightful news.

An egg yolk's second greatest virtue is its brain-charging abilities. The combination of choline, inositol and top-class protein helps nourish our mental and physical stamina. Dynamite fodder for the eggsam season - sorry. Other virtues include impressive levels of feel-good tryptophan, cancer-fighting selenium and calcium-loving vitamin D. A cracking concoction.

5 egg yolks
zest and juice of 1 large or
  2 small unwaxed lemons
5 tablespoons extra virgin
  coconut oil
5 tablespoons light agave,
  raw honey or brown rice
  syrup

Serves 4-8

Using a small saucepan on a low setting, gently heat all the ingredients. Make sure you are continuously whisking with a metal balloon beater - that's the whisky-looking implement usually reserved for beating egg whites.

When all the coconut oil has melted, keep a watch for little bubbles forming on the surface, telling you the mixture is getting hotter and hotter. By then you should notice the curd getting thicker. Test it by dipping the back of a spoon into it. If the curd coats the spoon, remove it from the heat. If it runs off, keep the curd over the heat until it thickens a little more.

Pour the lemon curd into pristine-clean jam jars or espresso cups. Serve with a simple spoon and a ravenous appetite.

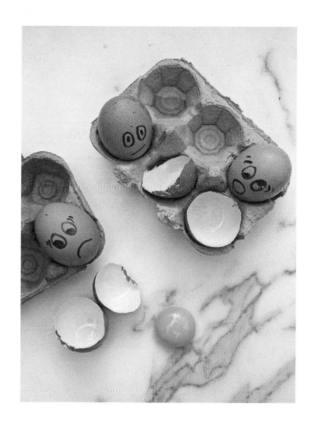

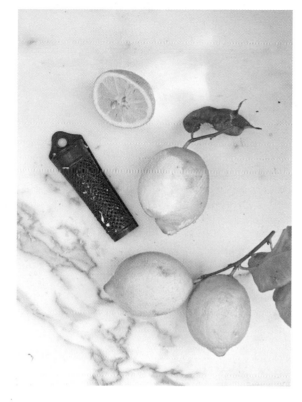

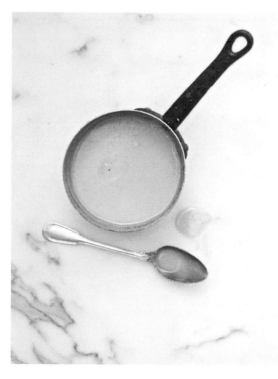

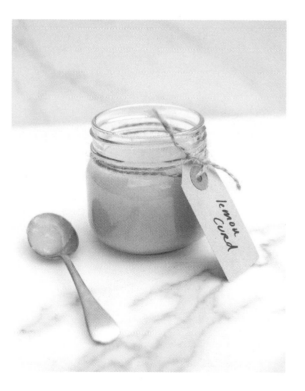

SAINTLY TREATS

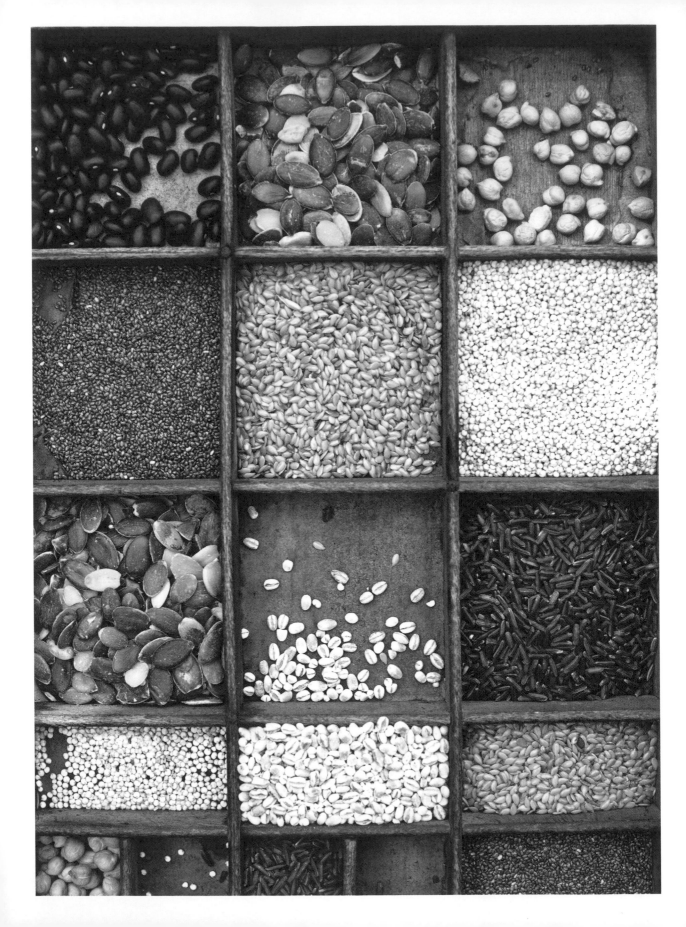

BIRCH SUGAR GRANOLA

≪≫≪≫≪≫≪≫≪≫≪≫≪≫

For the candida warriors and diabetics among us. My ode to xylitol is on page 17.

Fire up your oven to 170°C/150°C fan/340°F. Line two baking trays with good non-stick parchment (see page 201 in the resources section).

If your xylitol is rather grainy, you'll need to whizz it in a coffee grinder or high-speed blender until it looks more like fairy dust. Then scoop it into a large saucepan with the coconut oil and cinnamon. Let them relax together on a low heat for 5 minutes.

Once the oil has melted, add the oat and quinoa flakes. Parachute in your favourite nuts (I love hazelnuts and pecans for this recipe), a scattering of seeds and the sea salt flakes.

Whisk the egg whites (if using) in a spotlessly clean, dry bowl until soft and droopy. They don't need to stand in stiff peaks. Fold into the granola mix. I don't always do this - it depends on my mood. Egg whites help to make soft clusters in the granola, but if you prefer it dead crunchy, leave the egg whites out.

Spread the granola over your lined trays. Roast for 18-22 minutes, removing from the oven before the oats turn brown and bitter.

Leave to cool entirely before adding the goji berries, cacao nibs and coconut. They all tend to burn in the oven, so they're best left until last.

Store in a massive glass jar and your sleepy taste buds will backflip every morning when you catch sight of it.

under $^1/_2$ cup (100g) xylitol
1 cup (250ml) melted coconut oil
1 tablespoon ground cinnamon
2 cups (180g) oat flakes
1 cup (100g) quinoa flakes (or more oat flakes)
2 cups (150g) nuts, chopped
$^1/_2$ cup (70g) sunflower and pumpkin seeds
$^1/_2$ teaspoon sea salt flakes
3 egg whites (optional, to make clusters)
6 tablespoons goji berries
6 tablespoons raw cacao nibs
6 tablespoons desiccated coconut

Makes 25 portions

ACTIVATED NUTS

《》《》《》《》《》《》

Activated nuts sound like something you'd find in the front row of an ACDC concert. But they are in fact a fundamental snack in the vegan's pantry.

Many health enthusiasts insist on sprouting and drying nuts before using them in recipes. It is thought that an obstructive phytate layer on nuts can inhibit the proper breakdown of the nut's nutrition. There is some evidence to suggest that this phytic acid acts as an anti-nutrient and can complicate calcium's absorption, for example. I haven't seen satisfying scientific research to support this theory, but they sure do taste better! To get rid of this phytic layer, soaking in slightly salted water apparently helps.

On the other hand, food scientist Harold McGee believes salt extracts water-soluble vitamins and minerals like calcium into the water. He recommends always using the soaking water from beans when cooking them, for example. As you can see, this theory competes with the accepted wisdom of soaking nuts to improve nutrition. It's up to you to make the final decision: folklore versus science. I don't really do it, but here's a recipe just so you know how.

4 cups (400-450g) nuts
2 teaspoons fine sea salt

Makes 4 cups (400-450g)

Cover the nuts with fresh filtered water and the salt. Leave them to soak for 8 hours or overnight. Rinse and drain.

Spread them out on a baking tray and let them dry in a warm oven - I do this at 50°C/30°C fan/85°F or in a dehydrator - for 8-24 hours, until they are completely crisp. Pecans only take 8 hours, but Brazil nuts will take longer.

Prepared this way, nuts can be stored at room temperature for several months and used for any of the recipes throughout this book. They taste exceptionally good.

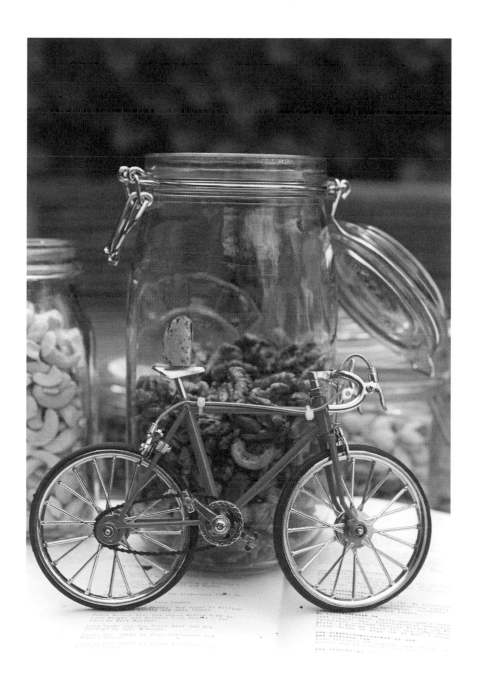

SAINTLY TREATS

TOASTED PECANS

《 》《 》《 》《 》《 》《 》

'I don't diet and exercise,' says three-time Olympian Derval O'Rourke, 'I eat and train'. Sage words from a seriously cool athlete. This is Derval's go-to snack. Be good to your body. You're the one who has to live in it.

1 cup (110g) pecans
2 tablespoons agave or maple
  syrup
pinch of sea salt flakes

Makes 10 portions

Whack up the oven to 160°C/140°C fan/325°F. Line a baking tray with baking parchment.

Spread the pecans across the lined tray and let them get giddy with the syrup and sea salt. You could also use a pinch of your favourite spice, such as ground star anise, garam masala, ground cinnamon or smoked paprika.

Pop the tray into your oven for 12–20 minutes. Toss the nuts on the tray halfway through the cooking time to prevent burning and tantrums.

Remove from the oven before the nuts turn too dark and give the pecans a decent chance of cooling before plundering the entire batch. The pecans are much crunchier and sweeter upon cooling.

Store in a jar and sprinkle onto porridge, salads and thirsty fingers throughout the week.

BANANA POPSICLES

«»«»«»«»«»«»

These ice pops are The Snazz. Great hunks of creamy banana with brittle chocolate and superfoods to nourish your little ones this summer. And at the same time gift Mum and Dad with 10 minutes of celestial silence. Air. Punch.

Frozen bananas will deliver a consignment of B vitamins to recharge our battery and smile dial. These chaps also house lots of potassium, an important mineral to help with hydration in the sun.

Chop each banana in half (not down the middle like a banana split). Insert a wooden ice lolly stick into the bottom of each half to make four banana popsicles. Place on a piece of non-stick parchment and freeze for 2 hours.

Meanwhile, slowly melt the chocolate and hazelnut butter (if using) in a bain-marie. This is basically a pot of simmering water, 2.5cm in depth, with a heatproof bowl sitting on top where a lid might otherwise have gone. The contents of the bowl will gently melt from the steam of the water underneath. The trick is not to let the water boil and don't let the bottom of the bowl touch the water underneath.

Dip the top of each frozen banana into the melted chocolate and return to the freezer for an extra 5 minutes to set. Alternatively, dip each frozen banana pop first into melted chocolate and then roll in finely chopped goji berries, chopped pistachios, chopped pumpkin seeds, raw cacao nibs, hemp seeds or bee pollen. Let your taste buds vote.

2 bananas, peeled
8 squares of dark or raw chocolate
1-2 tablespoons hazelnut butter (optional)

OPTIONAL COATING:
finely chopped goji berries, chopped pistachios, chopped pumpkin seeds, raw cacao nibs, hemp seeds or bee pollen

Makes 4 popsicles

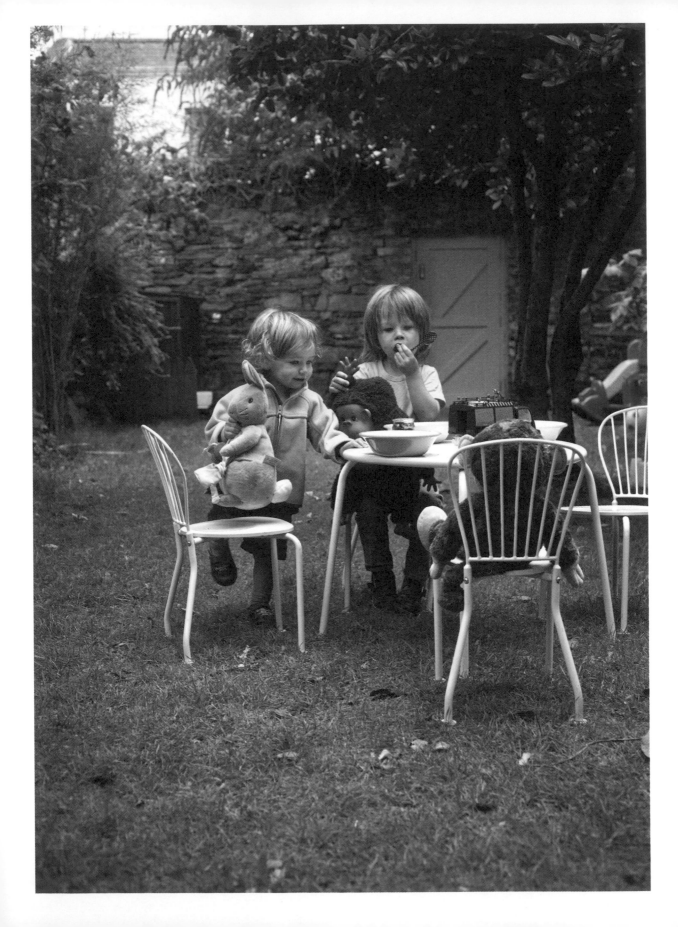

STRAWBERRY AND LIQUORICE ICE CREAM

《》《》《》《》《》《》《》《》《》《》《》《》《》《》

Think of strawberries as beauty bullets. Soaked with anti-inflammatory compounds, skin-plumping vitamin C and antioxidants, strawberries can help deter the pesky ageing process. And likely increase your chances of a Helen Mirren bikini moment. Make this ice cream and feel the vitamins dance towards your skin.

The key to this ice cream is using slightly more frozen banana than frozen strawberries, but 50:50 will still work beautifully. Before freezing the banana, peel and chop the flesh into small discs. Freeze on baking parchment, making sure each slice doesn't fraternise with its neighbour. Once they're frozen, you can store them in a large glass jar or bag and use as needed.

I buy great-value frozen strawberries at my local four-letter German supermarket, so I rarely bother freezing fresh ones. If you prefer to freeze fresh berries, follow the same route as the banana above.

Blend the frozen fruit with the liquorice on the highest setting you have. A Vitamix or OmniBlend will do this in 5 seconds; a regular blender will take 15 seconds. You'll need a splash of plant-based milk - I use oat milk for children's parties if there's someone with a nut allergy.

Scoop into pre-chilled tumbler glasses and tuck straight in. Leftovers don't refreeze very well. I doubt you'll hate me for it.

1 banana
big palmful of frozen
  strawberries
pinch of liquorice powder or
  1 bag of liquorice tea
a trickle of plant-based
  milk

Serves 1-3

Variations to play with if you're making this strawberry ice cream every summer afternoon:

• Fresh mint leaves from the garden

• 2.5cm chunk of frozen ginger, grated into the food processor bowl

• Chocolate chips

• 1 green cardamom pod, black seeds coaxed into the food processor bowl

• Raw honey or stevia, to sweeten

• 2 teaspoons of vibrant beetroot powder

• The flesh of 1 mango and some anti-inflammatory ground turmeric

• A touch of fresh basil and black pepper

• Tumble the juicy seeds from a passion fruit over a scoop of ice cream before serving

• Decorate with bee pollen

4

BORN AGAIN TRUFFLES

SWEETS TO LOVE THAT LOVE YOUR BODY BACK

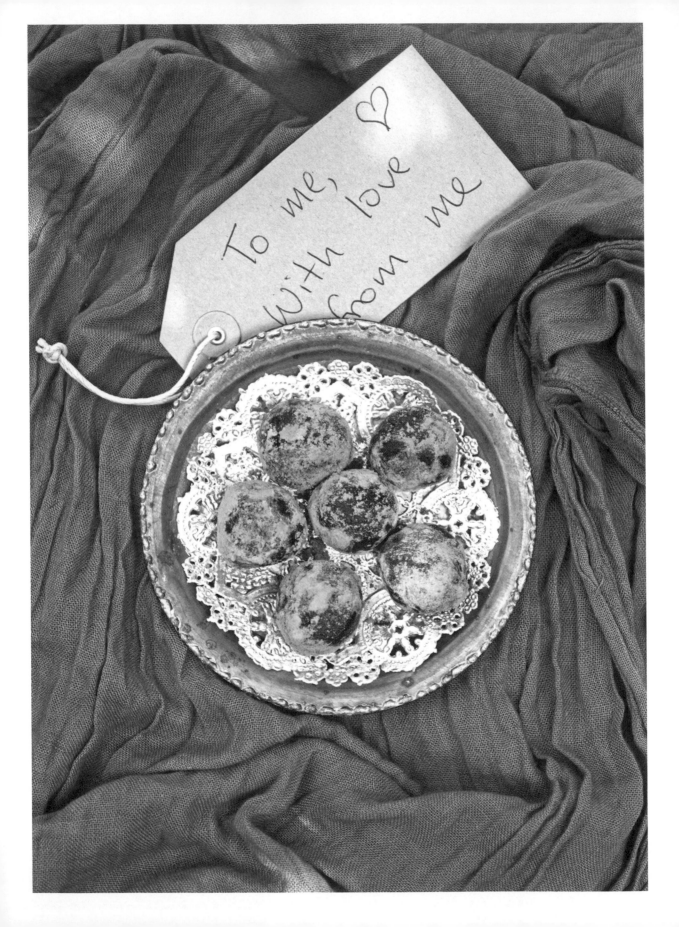

AMAZONTAN TRUFFLES

≈≈≈≈≈≈≈≈≈≈≈≈≈

Practically humming with energy, the sesame and chia seeds in this recipe will deliver a fleet of minerals to service your mojo. These seeds are also crammed with B vitamins to nourish frayed nerves and low batteries at a fraction of the price of a marriage counsellor. You're welcome.

Just two truffles will deliver 100% of your recommended daily allowance (RDA) of vitamin E. Ooh argh! This vitamin is hailed as one of the most powerful antioxidants in the fight against free radical damage (that's fancy speak for ageing skin). Think of vitamin E as the patron saint of Eternal Youth.

With a fork, beat the tahini, maple syrup, acai powder and a pinch of sea salt flakes together in a medium bowl until sumptuously glossy. Measure in the remaining ingredients and encourage them to rumba. This may take a bit of persuasion.

Take a cherry-sized ball of the mixture and roll it between the palms of your hands to form a soft truffle. Drop each one into cocoa powder and roll it around to coat it. Set on a cold plate. As soon as you've used up all the mixture (you should get 30 or so truffles), refrigerate them. Keep your thirsty fingers busy while the truffles set. One hour should do the trick.

There's no need to stick to acai powder in this recipe. Try ground ginger for a cheaper alternative or dust the truffles in beetroot powder for Barbie-loving toddlers.

¹/₄ cup (60ml) light or dark tahini
¹/₄ cup (60ml) maple syrup
2 tablespoons acai powder
pinch of sea salt flakes
¹/₂ cup (45g) milled chia seeds
4 tablespoons ground almonds
2 tablespoons cocoa or cacao powder, plus extra for dusting

Makes 30 truffles

MEGA RASPBERRY BOMBS

≈≈≈≈≈≈≈≈≈≈≈≈≈≈≈≈≈

I know they sound rather rude, but these mega raspberry bombs are in fact devastatingly tasty. Fresh raspberries won't work and dried ones are too expensive, but raspberry leaf tea gives an unimaginably delicious smack of sherbet. And no, they won't make your cervix dilate.

If you can't find milled sunflower and pumpkin seeds, just whizz enough of both seeds until they resemble fine breadcrumbs. I tend to use hemp powder in place of ground almonds for my boys' lunch boxes because of school nut policies. And if you don't have goji berries, no problem. I just used them to give the impression of raspberries flecked throughout the mixture.

3 raspberry leaf teabags
1 cup (120g) milled sunflower
  and pumpkin seeds
$^1/_2$ cup (50g) ground almonds
  or hemp seed powder
$^1/_3$ cup (50g) raisins
$^1/_3$ cup (85ml) maple or brown
  rice syrup
4 tablespoons light or dark
  tahini
2-3 tablespoons carob powder
2 tablespoons goji berries
$^1/_2$ teaspoon sea salt flakes

Makes 40 truffles

Tear the teabags open and pour the dried leaves into the bowl of a food processor. Blitz with the remaining ingredients until thoroughly socialised. You may need to scrape down the sides of the bowl as you go along.

Roll the dough into little bombs between the palms of your hands. Depending on the consistency of the tahini you used, the mixture might be dry or gooey. If it looks too wet to roll, add more milled seeds. If it looks too dry, try a touch more tahini. Let them set in the fridge for 2 hours.

These will keep for three weeks in the fridge or in the freezer for three months. Or three seconds in your hands.

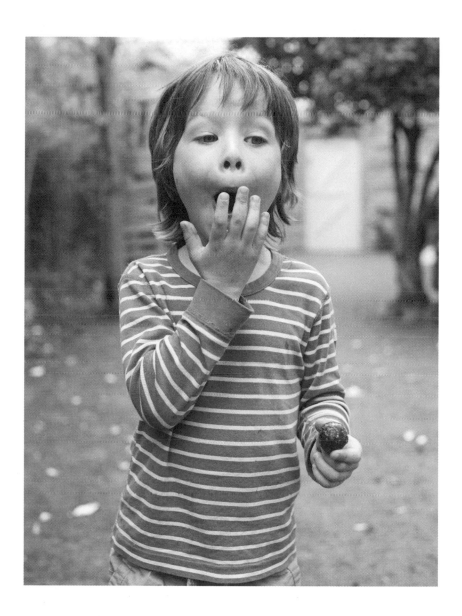

BORN AGAIN TRUFFLES

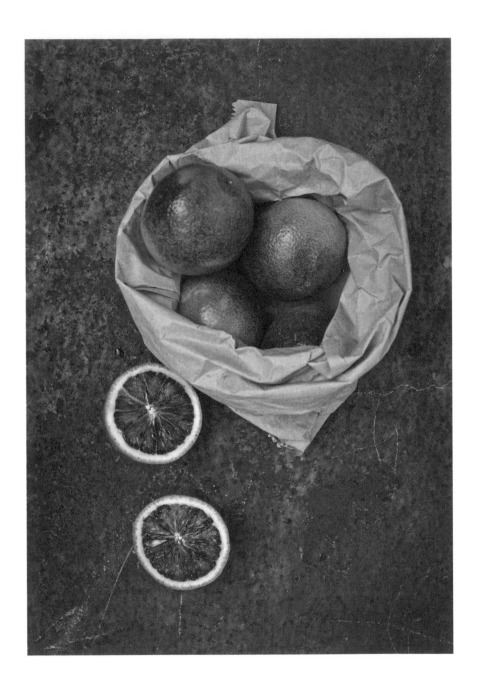

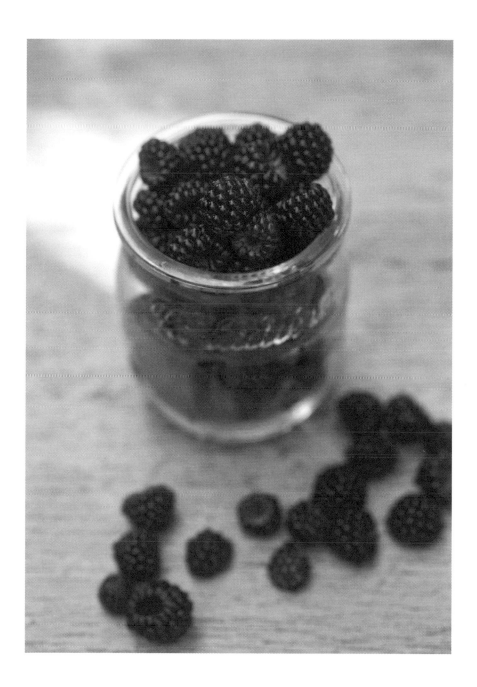

BORN AGAIN TRUFFLES

SPIRULINA GRENADES

≈≈≈≈≈≈≈≈≈≈≈≈≈≈

Mixed with water, spirulina powder looks and tastes like a fertile frog pond. Ascetic accessories are trending this season, so I predict spirulina will have a stonking good year. Whiff aside, this blue-green algae has enough nutrients to make blueberries whimper. Spirulina is the superhero of superfoods.

So what's all the fuss about? Spirulina has an impressive iron and amino acid profile, making it attractive to bench pressers and vegetarians. Why should you care? Because iron is vital for energy. This mineral helps manufacture haemoglobin in our red blood cells, which is responsible for ferrying oxygen around our bloodstream. Iron can also act as a fancy enzyme in the metabolic pathways that turn glucose into energy. That's fancy lingo for more go-go juice. This might help explain why a deficiency in iron can lead to fatigue and dizziness. Women are in greater need of iron than men due to our pesky cycle.

What else? Spirulina is also a useful source of B vitamins. Think B for Usain Bolt. B vitamins are the ones considered crucial for energy ignition. It's easy to see why athletic folk love this curious green powder.

These energy grenades are the best way to sneak this legendary water plant into your diet. After all, healthy eating should never sacrifice your taste buds.

16 Medjool dates, stones removed
2 tablespoons extra virgin coconut oil
2 tablespoons almond butter
1 tablespoon spirulina powder
1-2 teaspoons tamari soya sauce
1 tablespoon cocoa, lúcuma or maca powder, for dusting

Makes 20-30 truffles

Destone the Medjools before dropping them into a food processor. Add the coconut oil, almond butter, spirulina powder and tamari, saving the dusting for later. Whizz on a low speed until blended.

Using a teaspoon, mould the mix into teeny bonbons. Your hands will naturally become slippery, aiding the process. Expect to get 20 to 30 bonbons from the batch, depending on how many times the teaspoon fell into your mouth.

Chill for 12 hours before rolling the bonbons in the cocoa, lúcuma or maca powder. Any sooner, and the bonbon will drink up the coating.

You can find a video demo of this recipe on my YouTube channel. They're the original amazeballs.

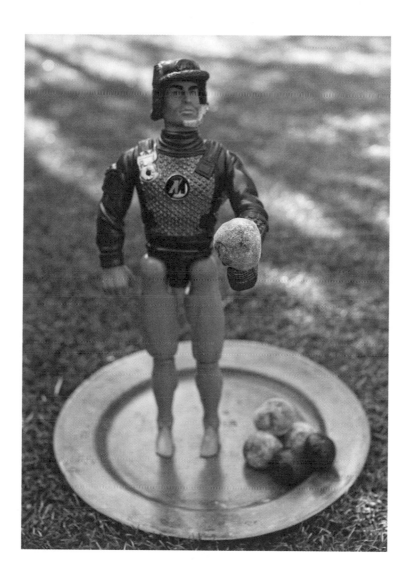

BORN AGAIN TRUFFLES

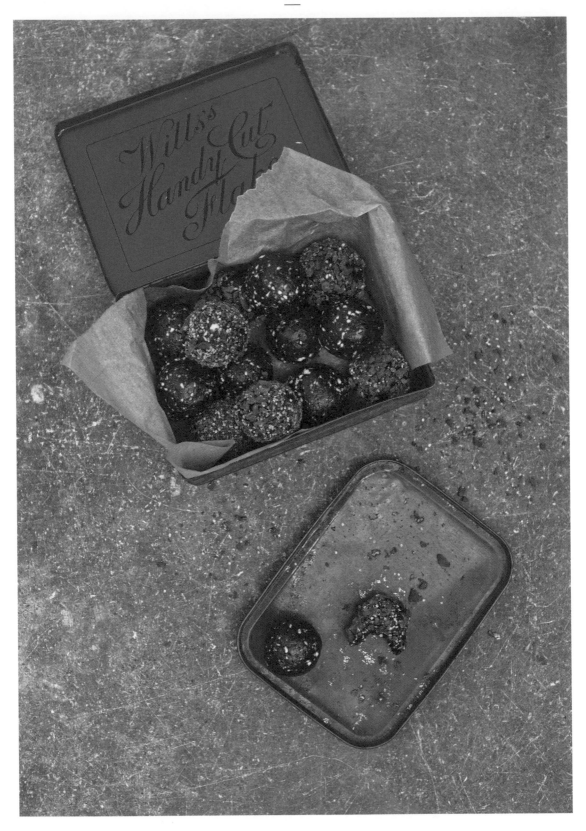

PEPPERMINT-LACED ENERGY BALLS

≈≈≈≈≈≈≈≈≈≈≈≈≈≈≈≈≈≈≈≈≈≈≈≈≈≈

*No need to straddle a packet of biscuits for your afternoon snack. When you
have these energy balls programmed into your kitchen's DNA, you'll feel the
health benefits faster than immediately.*

Blend all the ingredients except the gojies in a
food processor and whizz until it clumps together
in a large dough ball. One minute should be
about right. Taste and decide if it needs more
peppermint to mask the taste of spirulina. Too
much will taste like toothpaste, so watch out!

Make 20 golf ball-sized truffles or 30-40 smaller
ones by rolling some dough between your palms.
Place on a non-stick tray and chill until
relatively firm. Once set (about 30 minutes), roll
them in the bright red goji berry dust. Raw cacao
powder or desiccated coconut work well too, but
the racy red colour of gojies makes my eyes go
giddy up.

Store in the freezer and grab on the run. (With
special reverence to Chitra, my neighbour.)

1 ½ cups (225g) Medjool
  dates, stones removed
1 cup (140g) almonds
¼ cup (20-25g) cacao powder
3 tablespoons extra virgin
  coconut oil
1 tablespoon spirulina
  powder
1-2 teaspoons tamari
¼ teaspoon organic
  peppermint extract or 4
  drops of culinary-grade
  peppermint oil
3 tablespoons goji berries,
  very finely chopped

Makes 20-40 truffles

HEALTH BY CHOCOLATE

≈≈≈≈≈≈≈≈≈≈≈≈≈≈≈≈

What's the difference between cacao and cocoa, apart from pomposity? Cacao is a raw, unadulterated form of the chocolate bean, whereas regular cocoa has been heat treated and roasted for a longer shelf life. Cocoa is also much darker in colour than cacao. That's not to say one is good and the other is bad. Let's take a closer peek.

Cacao beans are grown inside rugby-shaped pods. Each pod contains dozens of moist beans, which must be dried under the hot sun before they are sold as beans. Their cracked, papery skins need to be removed at this point. To do this, the beans are shot against a wall at full force with a fan blowing on them. As the beans shatter and the skins come off, the fan blows the skins away and the nibs fall into a large container for collection. These nibs are crunchy, slightly bitter and malty. You can buy them raw in most health stores to decorate your morning bowl of porridge. The nibs are then cold pressed into a thick paste. The cacao butter is separated, while the remaining mass is dried to make raw cacao powder.

The production of cocoa is much the same, except the cacao beans are fermented and roasted first and the end product is further heat-treated.

Raw cacao will score higher on the antioxidant radar, helping to decoy the ageing process. But cocoa is much easier to source in shops, is half the cost and deeper in flavour. Which is more important? That's for you to decide.

1 tablespoon raw cacao nibs
sprinkle of sea salt flakes
1/3 cup (85ml) melted cacao
  butter
2 tablespoons maple syrup or
  agave (not coconut nectar)
1 tablespoon melted extra
  virgin coconut oil
4 tablespoons raw cacao or
  cocoa powder

Makes 16 truffles

Start by chilling your chocolate mould in the freezer. I use a silicone ice cube tray. Loosely sprinkle in the cacao nibs and a flurry of sea salt flakes.

Slowly melt the cacao butter in a bain-marie until you get 1/3 cup (85ml). A bain-marie is basically a pot of gently simmering water with a heatproof bowl sitting on top in place of the lid. The contents of the bowl will melt gradually from the steam of the water underneath. Just make sure the bottom of the bowl doesn't touch the simmering water.

Using a fork, whisk through the remaining ingredients, keeping the bowl warm to prevent it from seizing. Work at speed! Vite!

Pour into the moulds and place in the freezer for 10 minutes. Store in the fridge thereafter for up to six weeks. And send me some telepathic jubilation.

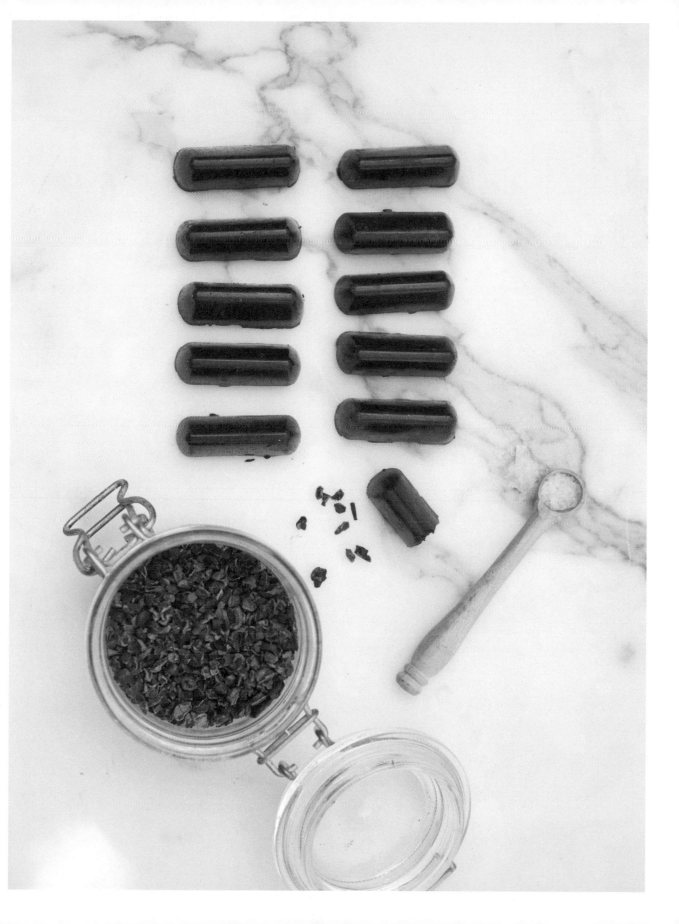

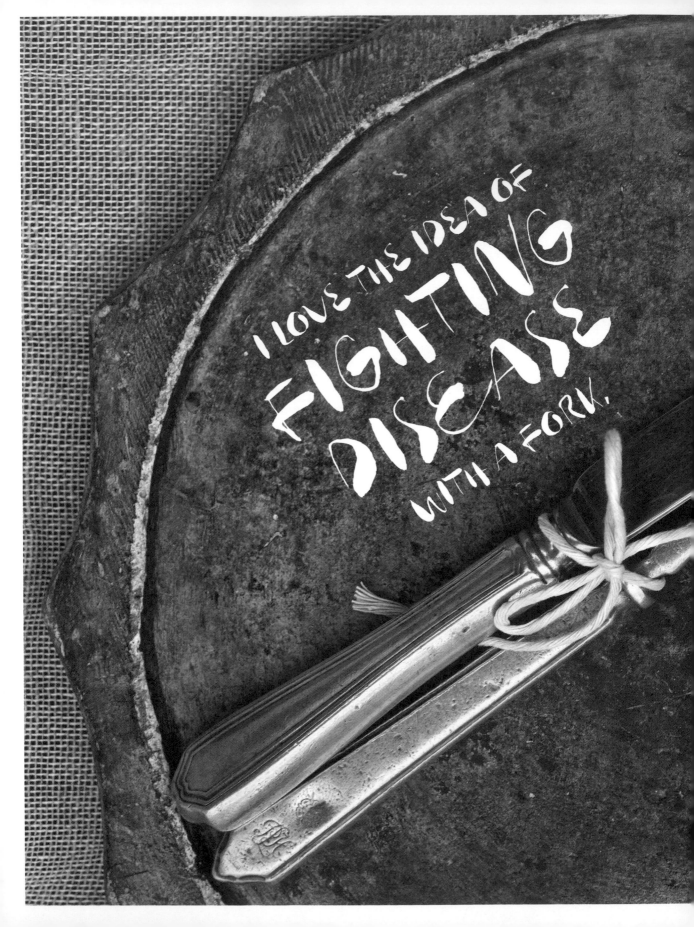

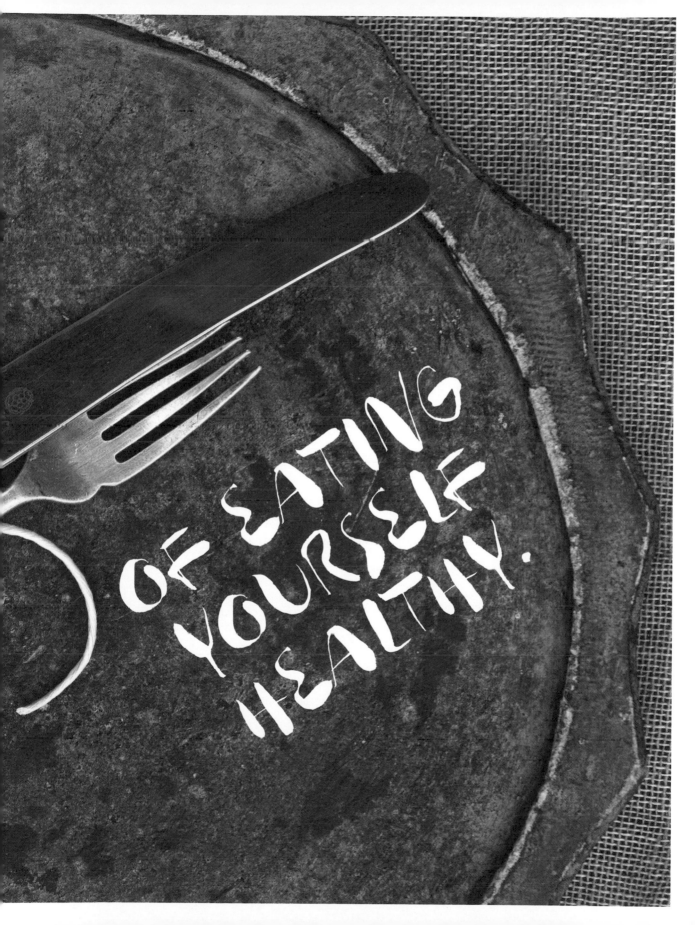

SEA SALTEASERS

≈≈≈≈≈≈≈≈≈≈≈

Meet your new friends, the Sea Salteasers, designed to tickle your tongue and your brain. Chia seeds are one of Mother N's best plant sources of omega-3 fuel. We need omega-3s to oil our network of synapses and our Sudoku skills.

Chia seeds can swell up to 10 times their own weight, making them a perfect choice for weight watchers because they can make us feel fuller for longer. Chia seeds are also a surprising source of bone-building boron and calcium. Not a bad choice for your pipes either.

These teeny-weeny seeds will seem like an extravagant addition to your weekly shopping bill - that is, until you inaugurate Sea Salteasers into your pantry. They are The Snazz. Besides, I rather fancy Michael Pollan's attitude towards his shopping list: 'It's better to pay the grocer than the doctor.'

6 tablespoons barley malt
  syrup
4 tablespoons light or dark
  tahini
1 teaspoon real vanilla
  extract
4 tablespoons milled chia
  seeds
4 tablespoons ground almonds
3 tablespoons cocoa powder
good pinch of sea salt flakes

Makes 30 truffles

Start by downloading a good podcast. You'll be locked to the kitchen counter rolling bonbons for 20 minutes.

Using a fork, beat the barley malt syrup, tahini and vanilla together in a saucepan over your lowest heat. As soon as the mix turns glossy and luscious, take it off the heat. Measure in the remaining ingredients and encourage them to fraternise. Tenacity is useful - malt is seriously sticky.

Taking a small cherry-sized ball of the mixture, roll it between the palms of your hands to form a sweetie. They'll feel fairly limp, but they'll firm up once chilled. You should get about 30 balls.

Store them in the fridge or freezer and plunder at will. You might need to briefly reshape them before serving to someone you're trying to impress. And boy oh boy, will they work.

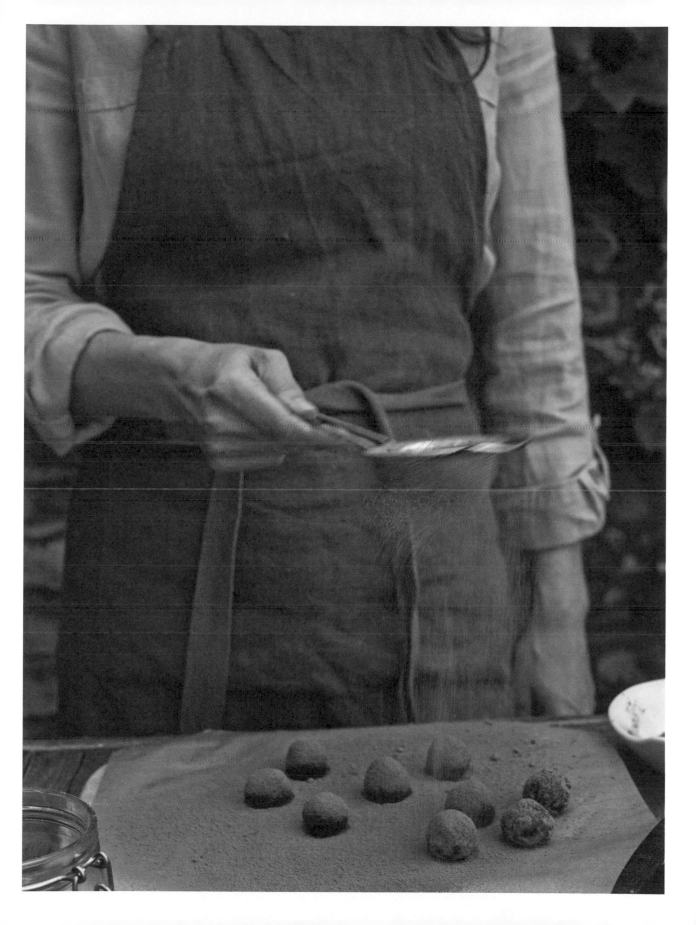

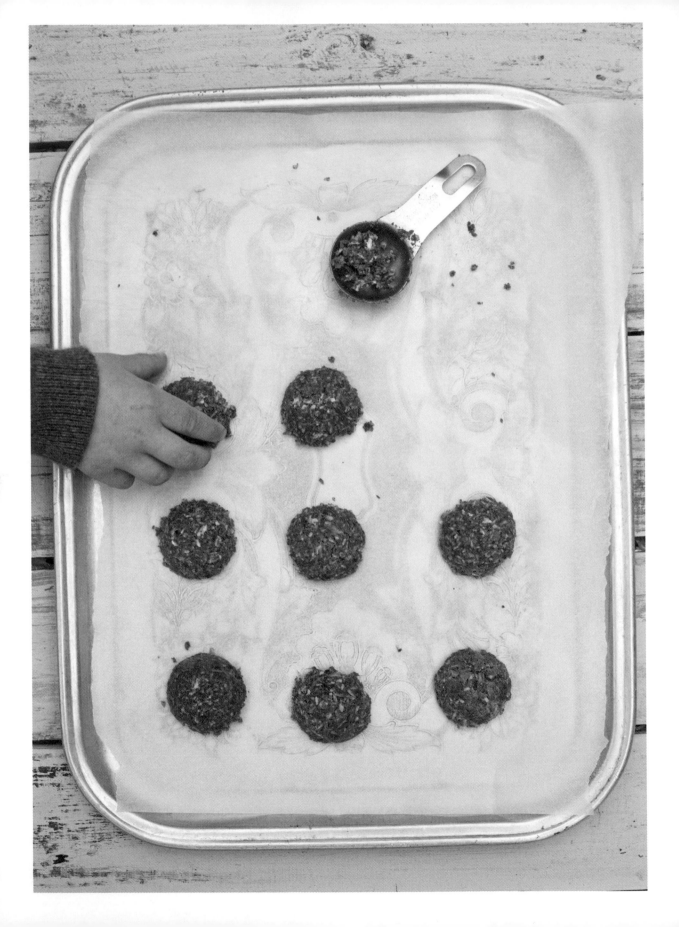

ACAI AND BEETROOT MACAROONS

≈≈≈≈≈≈≈≈≈≈≈≈≈≈≈≈≈≈≈≈≈≈

Acai (pronounced ass-sigh-ee) is the latest nutrient-dense Brazilian bomb. Deep purple in colour, acai berries may appear like swollen, egotistical blueberries at first glance, but in fact they are twice as potent - and five times as expensive.

You can expect to taste a confusing hybrid of blackberry and chocolate. This makes acai a brilliant partner for fruity smoothies or hot cocoa. In truth, this berry's nutritional purchase excites me more than its weird flavour. It's full of heart-healthy plant sterols, inflammation-reducing anthocyanins and boisterous antioxidants. That's a jolly fine combo. No, acai won't lower cholesterol like some dodgy websites promise, nor will this superfood cure pram brain. It is, however, another nourishing berry to introduce to your culinary playground, but not necessarily your medicine cabinet. And these macaroons certainly beat snacking on boiled sweets any day.

Psyche yourself up in the kitchen before starting. Look for Rodrigo y Gabriela and crank up the volume. Trust me, their rhythm will transfer to your fingertips.

Line a breadboard with parchment paper, then blitz all the ingredients in a food processor until it clumps together. My processor usually takes 30 seconds to do this.

Scoop out a small piece of dough and form it into a mini macaroon. Place on the parchment paper and repeat until all the dough is gone. I use my special metric tablespoon that's curved like a mini falafel scoop. The dough slides out beautifully and results in uncharacteristically professional-looking confectionary. Expect to get about 15 mini macaroons from the batch.

Freeze until solid, then transfer to your refrigerator.

1 ½ cups (120g) desiccated coconut
4 tablespoons raw honey (or raw light agave if diabetic)
3 tablespoons extra virgin coconut oil
2 tablespoons coconut flour
2 teaspoons beetroot powder
1 teaspoon acai berry powder
1 teaspoon vanilla extract or pure powder
squeeze of lemon or lime juice
pinch of sea salt flakes

Makes 15 mini macaroons

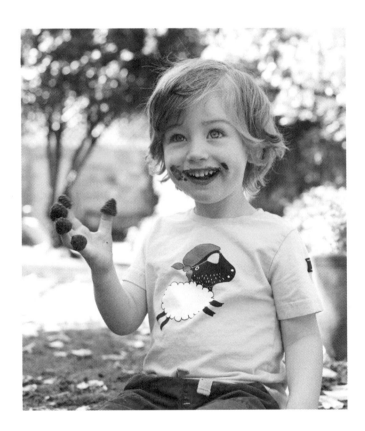

ONLINE RESOURCES

WHERE CAN YOU BUY ALL THIS WEIRD-SOUNDING STUFF?

Your local health food store will stock all the dried ingredients listed. If something is missing from their shelves, just ask! In my experience, health food stores are always eager to satisfy personal requests and explore new trends.

If frequenting a health food store sounds about as appealing as necking a glass of sneeze, here are a few helpful online resources that I use to bulk buy. Hope it helps.

www.wholefoodsmarket.com
A phenomenal whole foods store that stocks every single ingredient featured in this cookbook and much, much more. From quirky freeze-dried passion fruit to sprouted buckwheat granola, Whole Foods is a kingdom of goodness. Every time I visit their stores in London or Glasgow, I almost combust with excitement. It's worth the flight.

www.linwoodshealthfoods.com
If you don't have your own coffee grinder to finely mill seeds, Linwoods does a top-class range. They also offer free delivery of freshly milled seeds within Ireland and the UK. Essential for recipes such as Secret Agent Gingerbread (page 155) and Mega Raspberry Bombs (page 182).

www.realfoods.co.uk
For all those new flours filling your shopping list, such as teff and sorghum. Real Foods is a brilliant online grocer, providing absolutely everything you need for a whole food pantry.

www.alchemyjuice.ie
Order a supply of cold-pressed juices, dried kale, quinoa rolls, brainiac brownies, raw chocolate – the lot. Or drop in to them on Grafton Street in Dublin city centre. Their menu is free from dairy, cane sugar, wheat and gluten. Grab a nut milk bag while you're there too.

www.iswari.net and www.otesuperfoods.com
All manner of superfoods, from bee pollen to cacao butter, delivered to your doorstep. Saves a lot of lugging and chugging, especially if you use vats of coconut oil. Look out for Iswari's gluten-free sprouted oat flakes, which are much cheaper online than in store. At the time of going to print, Of The Earth (OTE) is one of the only stockists of yacón syrup.

**www.organicsupermarket.ie and
www.waitrose.com**
Home delivery of organic goodness and
dried staples if you're not close to a
health food store in Ireland and the
UK. Both sell the If You Care brand of
baking parchment, which is the best
non-stick parchment on the market.

www.brookfield.farm
You'll find local varieties of raw honey
in all good health food stores and
delis, but Brookfield Farm is special.
Their methods are biodynamic and
cold filtered. You can even buy a hive
timeshare - for real!

www.synerchikombucha.com
When you couldn't be arsed making your
own, Laura Murphy brews raw effervescent
kombucha tea. I dig.

www.josephjoseph.com
British measuring cups are essential,
as the American cup is only 237ml.
Joseph Joseph also does colourful, funky
digital scales, silicone spatulas and
bowls with pouring lips for making nut
milks. Delivery free to your home or
office.

www.nealsyardremedies.com
For culinary-grade essential oils like
peppermint for the After Eight Dinner
Party Torte on page 107 or bergamot for
the Earl Grey Chocolate Tartlets on page
101.

www.ifyoucare.com
The best baking parchment on the market.
It saves on sticking and tantrums.
Materials are unbleached, naturally
derived and FSC certified.

www.realseeds.co.uk
Organic high-quality seeds posted to
your door. Grow your own edible flowers
to decorate celebration cakes. Or get
your kale on.

www.amazon.co.uk
Springform tins for all the tarts in
this book: 20cm, 18cm, 15cm and 6cm. Nut
milk bags. OmniBlends and Nutribullets.

www.thatprotein.com
Really fabulous plant-based protein
powders to sneak into your children's
meals and Weetabix every morning. I use
them in the Mega Raspberry Bombs (page
182) to change things up a little or
sprinkle them into Camu Camu Cookies
(page 140), chocolate tortes and
smoothies.

www.keennutbutter.com
I buy great big 1kg tubs of almond
butter from Irish company Keen and use
it for spreading, dunking and baking.
The best range of nut butters in
Europe, no kidding! The hazelnut one
is an excellent choice for newbies and
children starting out on their healthy
pilgrimage.

www.theculturedclub.com
Everything you need to start fermenting
your own green tea and coffee, including
the 'mother' or 'scoby'. Check out their
events page, 'Fermentation across the
nation'. This gal has a groove of her
very own, and you won't want to miss a
beat.

**www.ballybrado.com
and www.dunanyflour.com**
Peerless organic flours, grown, dried,
milled and packaged locally. Mainly
whole wheat, rye and oats.

www.drcoys.ie
Suppliers of stevia Erylite and coconut
flour.

www.optica.ie
I don't know if you've noticed, but my
specs are delicious. This is where I
shop.

INDEX

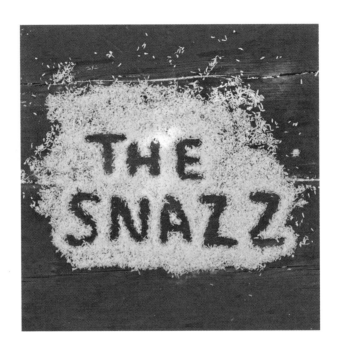

PRAISE FOR SUSAN JANE WHITE'S FIRST COOKBOOK,
THE EXTRA VIRGIN KITCHEN

'I can see why Susan Jane is a No 1 bestseller in Ireland. Brilliant approach to wholefood shop ingredients. Such a practical book.' **Joanna Blythman**

'This book is packed with naughty flavoured healthy food designed by the queen of guilt-free gobbling.' **Victoria Smurfit**

'Do you and your body a favour – read this book. Susan Jane White knows what's good for you and it doesn't hurt that she writes like a dream.' **Róisín Ingle, *The Irish Times***

'Her recipes seem like some delicious, illicit sin.' ***Irish Independent***

'If anyone ever needed proof that super-healthy food makes a huge difference to your energy levels, immune system and general vitality, then one look at the ever-effervescent Susan Jane White would tell you everything you need to know.' **Rachel Allen**